ACKNOWLED

Much like a pregnancy, this book had a long gestation period. I began thinking about it when pregnant with my daughter, but needed some time and space to sort it out. I also had a lot of help in bringing this book to light, and I hope I haven't forgotten anyone who needed to be thanked. To all my family, friends and acquaintances who had faith in this book, if I have left out your names, it is inadvertently.

Thank you to the six brave women who participated in my interviews. You took a chance on a pregnancy after a loss, which is a very brave step indeed. You also took a chance with me, agreeing to share your fears, joys, sorrows, excitement and hearts. This book would not be what it is without your contribution, and for that I am immensely grateful.

To all the people who gave feedback on my writing. In research circles, this is called member checking, and I am so glad you were there to provide your insights and thoughts on how to turn my initial drafts into something a person would actually want to read. Thank you.

To Dr. Graeme Smith, MD, PhD, FRCSC. Thanks for taking time to read through much of this book and providing your feedback and insight. And thanks for being with me through three pregnancies, and for not being afraid to show your grief when things went wrong and your joy when things went right. If EBP truly is the best research evidence, patient preferences AND clinical expertise, I was very glad to have your clinical expertise throughout.

Thanks also go to Corina Koch McLeod, for advice on editing and publishing and the world of writing. This book wouldn't exist were it not for your wise words, and your faith in my abilities. Thank you for being my friend.

Thanks to my wonderful editor, Carla Douglas, who always seemed to know what I wanted to say, even if I was not as elegant as I could have been in saying it. You helped sort out my thoughts and ramblings and made them beautiful and coherent.

To the delightful Kellie Wright, my book designer. These beautiful graphics, stunning cover design and glorious fonts are all her idea!

For my three awesome research assistants: Shona Macinnes, Craig Faucette, Roop Sandhu. The job of a research assistant is not always easy, but you saved my bacon. This book wouldn't exist without you.

To Lindsay Henke, Francesca Cox, Lori Mullins Ennis, Tova Gold, Beth Morey and the awesome writers at Still Standing Magazine and Pregnancy After Loss Support. You inspire me.

To my parents, for teaching me that girls can do anything. Anything.

To my children, Nate, Sam, Rebecca, Alexander. Nate and Sam, we miss you every day. Rebecca and Alexander, you will always be my greatest accomplishment. Every moment I spend with you is treasured, even if there are days I yell at you to pick up your toys. Again.

Last, but certainly not least, thanks go to my husband Michael White, for believing that I wasn't crazy, when everyone else was trying to tell me I was. For going against everything your New England sensibilities have taught you and wearing your heart on your sleeve, especially for all your feedback on the chapter for Dads. Thank you for loving me. In our first pregnancy, you wrote something special on our copy of What To Expect..., that "together we would cope with all the surprises". Somehow, we did. I couldn't have done any of this without you, and I wouldn't want to.

TABLE OF CONTENTS

FOREWORD

After a perfectly healthy nine-month pregnancy, my husband and I arrived at the hospital on a cold Minnesota December dawn. I was in labour, ready to welcome our first child into this world, only to be told, "I'm sorry. There is no heartbeat." Our lives were forever changed in that moment, when the doctor uttered the most devastating words a parent could ever hear. Our innocence was broken, our parenthood lost, and our daughter, Nora, was stillborn that afternoon.

Nora was a beautiful baby, with jet-black hair and a heart-shaped face that I fear one day I will forget. The hour we spent with her was both the most brutal and most beautiful 60 minutes of my life. How I wish I could have lived in that moment for a lifetime. When she left my arms for eternity that afternoon, a part of me left this earth forever with her too.

The grief of losing Nora was more than I believed I could ever bear. No words describe the weight of sadness that encompasses you in the days that follow the death of your child. The future, once filled with hope and possibility, had crumbled around us. Darkness was all we could see. As much as I yearned for Nora and could never replace her, the longing to be a parent to a living child still tugged at my heart.

In April of the following year, our heads and hearts aligned. We had reached a place in our grief where the desire to parent a living child outweighed the fear of losing another baby. We started to try again. In September we found ourselves pregnant with baby number two, due in March. The next nine months were the most emotionally challenging months of my life, full of fear and joy living side by side. We had no reason to believe in hope, but we held onto it anyway. At the same time, fears paralyzed me daily. I would whisper to the baby growing inside of me, "Please stay! Please stay!" and then pray to my dead daughter, "Please let me keep this one." We were lucky. Our baby did stay, and we got to keep her. Zoe was born healthy and alive 15 months after her older sister had died.

Pregnancy after loss is by far is the hardest thing I have ever done after surviving the death of my own child. During my pregnancy after loss I yearned for a book to walk me through this journey of grief and joy. I needed a guidebook, written by a mentor who had been there before me, handing me a map with the paths to surviving the nine-month journey of pregnancy after loss. Most of all I needed the hope offered from other courageous mamas' stories, how they gave birth to life instead of death.

With one in four pregnancies ending in miscarriage and one in 160 pregnancies ending in stillbirth, I thought that certainly a book like this existed! But it didn't, until now. Joy at the End of the Rainbow is the book for which I so desperately yearned. It's the What to Expect When You Are Expecting after a loss. Amanda Ross-White beautifully pours love into this week-by-week guidebook, walking the reader through what one might encounter during a pregnancy that follows a loss. She takes us into the worlds of six courageous mamas and gives us hope by following them through their pregnancies after loss. A dedicated researcher, Amanda combines her personal experience with evidence-based research into creating this much-needed book for the mom pregnant again after a loss.

Through Joy at the End of the Rainbow, Amanda Ross-White will be with you through your journey of pregnancy after loss--starting from the early stages of trying to conceive again, continuing on week-by-week through each trimester through the birth of your subsequent child and even into the postpartum period. A courageous mama herself, she will be your mentor and guide, continuously give you hope that through this pregnancy you, too, will give birth to life.

Lindsey Henke, Founder, Pregnancy After Loss Support (PALS)
February, 2017

Joy at the End of the Rainbow

1

INTRODUCTION
Who Am I and Why am I Writing this Book?

When I was in my fourth pregnancy, I needed a book that spoke to me. A book that addressed my fears and anxieties in a realistic way, without being patronizing. Most pregnancy books are filled with wonderful information, but they are written for the first-time mom. The woman who is thrilled to be pregnant and cannot wait for the next stage in her life. They were not written with women like me in mind—women who had been down this road before, but who had no living baby to show for it.

As a medical librarian, I was able to do my own research. I knew that there was not a book like this, and that research into coping through a pregnancy after a loss was scarce. I also knew that there was a great need for this kind of book, because there were far too many women like me. According to the World Health Organization, there are an estimated 33,000 perinatal deaths in North America each year [1]. This figure does not include miscarriages, the exact number of which is hard to determine. Everywhere I went, people confessed their own losses to me, or the losses of someone they knew. Even though I felt incredibly alone, there were many women who had made this journey before me. This book is intended for women who are brave enough to try again after a devastating loss.

My story begins in 2007, when my husband and I could not believe our good fortune. We were expecting not just one baby, but two! Recently married, we were eager to start our new family. My husband was over 40 and, at 29, I was the average age for first-time moms in Canada. We had great jobs and a house of our own. Everything seemed to have been right for us to begin the next stage in our lives. We never thought we could have twins, so that came as a shock, but we embraced the idea quickly, with all the extra work (and expense!) it would involve. It was a thrilling time. Our lives began to revolve around doctor's appointments, ultrasound appointments, prenatal classes, and all the shopping and prepping that modern pregnancy in North American life includes. Naturally, we bought a copy of What to Expect When You're Expecting. We charted my symptoms, carefully followed the diet plan, and read every page at least 10 times. There was joy in those nine months, knowing our lives would be forever changed. It was fun. We also bought a book for parents of multiples, thrilled about the special challenges involved in raising twins. The book had a couple of pages about what can go wrong, but that was it. Even though we knew there were risks, and knew that monozygotic (also called identical) twins were riskier, we did not let that dampen our enthusiasm. It did not even cross our minds. But, at 36 weeks and five days, the worst happened.

One Saturday morning, while my husband was out shopping for a second crib, I realized that I had not felt the baby move in some time. Exactly how long I could not say for certain, because I was busy that morning: I was cleaning the house, talking on the phone, continuing with life as normal. I initially thought they were sleeping, or had moved lower into my birth canal to get ready to come out. By the time my husband got back, I was in a panic. At first he was rather annoyed because I had been very stressed - the day before. He thought I was being overly anxious. But my mother-in-law told him not to dismiss my fears and to take me to hospital.

We went straight to the labour and delivery unit. The nurse came to check for a heartbeat, but she could not find one. She went to get the charge nurse. Again, the charge nurse could not find one, so she went to get the resident. The resident said she wanted to take a look on the ultrasound machine. I would have to move from the examination area, where they had all the beds set up in a row, to another room. That is when I knew they were taking me away so I would not upset everyone else. I could hear the charge nurse paging the chief OB/GYN, too, so I knew it was something the resident was not prepared to deal with on her own.

As soon as the chief OB/GYN confirmed there was no heartbeat, I became an automaton. No emotion, no feeling. I had mentally left the room. My husband cried and I just patted his head, unable to comfort him. The doctor recommended induction instead of a cesarean section because it would be better for future pregnancies. I wanted to be induced, too, because I wanted to know what labour felt like. I wanted to feel the contractions like all the normal mothers. When the anesthesiologist came to give me an epidural, he explained all the adverse effects:

"You could experience paralysis, even death, although the likelihood of that happening is the same as being struck by lightning twice." I remember thinking that I would not consider death to be an adverse effect. After nine hours of labour, my boys were born. I did not come out of my stupor until three days later, after the memorial service. That was when I finally realized that I was not going to bring them home.

We named our twins Nathaniel and Samuel. At first, we were not sure we wanted to name them, or if we should "save" the names for a future baby, but the nurse convinced us that these were their names. I am so glad she spoke up. We had pictures taken and impressions made of their hands and feet. We kept a lock of hair from each of them and a keepsake box with some clothing, blankets, and a teddy bear. These items are now some of my most treasured possessions. We were right on one count: Our lives have been forever changed.

Fast-forward some six months, and my husband and I were still deeply grieving, but desperately wanted to be pregnant again. Each month seemed to taunt us as we tried and failed, and the grief was renewed as we went through each monthly fertility window with no success. Finally, I found myself pregnant and nervously waiting to get through those precious 12 weeks.

The morning of a big presentation at work, and the Friday before my first Mother's Day, I was prepping in the bathroom of the conference centre. I was making sure my hair was brushed, that there was nothing between my teeth, no obvious flaws in my clothing . . . and I went into the stall to find the worst was happening again. I was having a miscarriage. A colleague raced me to the emergency room, knowing that there likely was not anything they could do. I still hoped that there was a heartbeat. I hoped I was mistaken, that this baby would not be lost, that this baby could be saved. The emergency room doctor was not as gentle as the obstetricians who delivered the bad news when my sons died. He made a joke about not being all that proficient with an ultrasound machine, and said he could not find a heartbeat, that I should go home and take it easy that weekend, then follow-up with my obstetrician on Monday. I was devastated. Intellectually I knew that an estimated one in three pregnancies ends in a miscarriage. Despite that, I believed that, given my previous loss, I would be rewarded with a baby. It was just too cruel to acknowledge that people lose more than one pregnancy. The grief began anew, now added to by new anxieties for future pregnancies. If I could lose two in a row, it seemed far too possible that I would lose yet another. The cycle began again.

In January of 2009, I was pregnant for the third time. This time I went straight to my high-risk obstetrician, the same one I had seen for my twins. This time I insisted on early ultrasounds. I was rewarded for all this vigilance with another pregnancy loss. This miscarriage was slightly earlier than the last one, 10 weeks instead of 12. It was just as devastating. As I watched women all around me get pregnant, have their babies, get pregnant again, have second babies, and so on, it seemed they were taunting me, making a mockery of my troubles. Well-meaning friends gave the most useless advice, "just relax," which implied that stress had caused me to miscarry. "There must have been something wrong." As if that would make me feel better. "It will happen." Again, as if no woman had ever been infertile. I was exhausted from the constant roller coaster of monthly cycles, where my moods reflected whether I was in the two-week waiting period of ovulation to period, or the two-week anticipation window of period to the next ovulation. I continued to mourn my sons each and every day, while simultaneously feeling the pain of losing the children I was afraid I would never have.

Then finally it happened. In March of 2009 I became pregnant yet again. We heard a heartbeat in the high-risk obstetrician's office at just six weeks. I had friends through support groups ready to help me every step of the way. Through the constant anxiety, fear, and watchful waiting of a subsequent pregnancy, my daughter was born. In 2011, we tried again for a baby. Again, this was a high-risk pregnancy, initially based on my history of pregnancy loss, but also because I developed pneumonia at the beginning of the third trimester. Pneumonia in pregnancy is serious, and I required a ventilator and spent 10 days in hospital with a collapsed lung, five of them in intensive care. I do not remember much of the experience, but it was painful, frightening, and difficult, especially for my husband, who had to be my decision-maker and spent time shuffling back and forth from my hospital bedside to the house, where our two-year-old daughter was asking questions about where mommy had gone. Fortunately, my son and I were both healthy by the time he was born in May of 2012.

For some of you, this story may resonate because it is all too similar to your own experience. However, a word of caution about this book: There are as many stories of pregnancy loss as there are pregnancies. This book is for all of you. Some of you will have had multiple losses, as I did. Some of you will have had early losses, at nine, 10, 11 weeks pregnant. Some of you will have late losses, at term, or post-term. Some of you may have had a cause found for your loss: gestational diabetes, strep infection, cord accident. Some of you are dealing with the anxiety of having no known cause for your loss. Some of you have even had to make the painful decision to terminate your pregnancy because your baby's condition was incompatible with life. Some of you got pregnant easily, some spent years on fertility treatments. Some of you lost your babies as teenagers, some of you as your biological clock ticked loudly in your ears.

For this reason, I have found a few friends along the way, people who have lost their babies in circumstances different from my own, who can help provide some insight into how their own experience can benefit you. Everyone used their own coping mechanisms to survive the next pregnancy. Some found help in their religious faith, others through art or music therapy, some from support groups both "in real life" and online. Wherever you find yourself on your pregnancy journey, I am hoping that you can take something from this text to help you. Feel free to discard any advice that does not fit your situation, and always, always remember that this book is not a replacement for medical advice. Talk to your doctor or midwife to see if anything in this book applies to you.

Also, because I am a medical librarian, I care deeply about using the best available medical evidence. While pregnancy after a loss is not well studied, I have taken what research is available to inform this book. Here I hope you will find a useful combination of medical evidence about pregnancy stages and concerns, written through the lens of someone who has been there before, someone whose anxiety and fear are rooted in her previous experience and who finds that all those other pregnancy guides do not quite work for her. Wherever you are in your journey, I wish you peace, and I hope you can use what you find here to make each step just a little easier. You are not alone.

A Note to Medical Professionals

As I mentioned above, I happen to be a patient who also has a day job. I work at Queen's University as a medical librarian, specifically in the School of Nursing, where I work with my nurse colleagues on systematic reviews. Originally, I had planned on writing a systematic review for the Joanna Briggs Institute on this topic, but before I had an opportunity to publish it, I got scooped. Twice [2, 3]! Not wanting to see my hard work go to waste, it seemed logical that I use the research to write a book for patients. Whenever I am asked what exactly librarians do, I describe my job like this:

Librarians connect people to information. And that is exactly what you will find in this book. If you have any questions or concerns about my research methodology or about my understanding of the research that informs this book, please contact me and I will do my best to update it for future editions. There is a complete bibliography at the end of this book. As a professional, if you find this book useful, I encourage you to write an information prescription for your patients. Physicians often take for granted that patients are comfortable seeking information online, although for a variety of reasons, that is not always the case. Directing your patients to quality information through an information prescription can be a useful way to start the conversation and ensure that patients are engaged in the shared decision-making process from an informed, evidence-based perspective.

2

TRYING AGAIN
Medical Concerns

With some exceptions, there are very few medical concerns you need to consider when it's time to try again. When it comes to making the decision, ultimately the only thing that matters is whether you and your partner feel ready. It is a deeply personal decision that you need to consider carefully, taking into account your unique situation. Many doctors will recommend waiting until your periods have returned to some regularity, which is likely at least six weeks and possibly even 12 weeks after you've given birth. This is partly because when the date of your last menstrual period is known, it is much easier to tell when you conceived. If you had an autopsy and genetic testing done, you may want to wait until the results are known, and this can take upwards of six weeks, sometimes longer.

Another medical consideration concerns the type of birth you had. If you had a cesarean birth, having another baby in less than a year's time often means the doctor will not want you to try for a vaginal birth. However, neither the Royal College of Obstetricians and Gynecologists (UK) or the American College of Obstetricians and Gynecologists indicate in their guidelines that this is a problem [4, 5].

Your age and your partner's age are also considerations for trying again. Age affects fertility for both men and women, so even if you are still under 35, if your partner is older, this should be considered. You will likely have an appointment with your doctor or midwife around six weeks after you gave birth, so it is a good time to talk about your plans for trying again, even if you do not yet feel ready. Some obstetricians recommend waiting up to six months or more before trying again, although much of this does not appear to be due to medical concerns [6, 7]. It is largely based on WHO recommendations, which looked at birth spacing outcomes in both healthy pregnancies and stillbirths (but not miscarriages), and included many studies done in lower, and lower-middle-income countries [8].

Psychological Concerns

Psychological concerns are a whole other issue. Many women report feeling a physical ache in their arms, so great is their commitment to having another child. Historically, professionals even called babies born after the death of a child "replacement children." We all know that this is not true. No child can ever replace one that has been lost. More recently, professionals have called these babies "penumbra children," because penumbra means "partially shaded area." [9, 10] The idea behind this term is that these babies are born in the shadow of their older siblings who died. I find it interesting that they use the term penumbra, meaning partially shaded, and not umbra, which means fully shaded. With a penumbra, some light is still coming through, which I find a beautiful analogy. A lot of mothers prefer to call their babies born after a loss "rainbow children," suggesting that after a rainstorm of tears there is still the beauty of the rainbow to look forward to. Whatever analogy you choose for your next pregnancy, there is no denying that it will be different. You will be anxious, you will feel the need to protect your heart from more hurt, you will still be grieving.

Grieving is hard work. It is exhausting, both mentally and physically. People who are depressed and grieving often have a hard time getting out of bed in the morning, and find themselves going back to bed, or at least to the couch, early in the evening. When you do sleep, it can be restless and of poor quality. You wake up just as exhausted as you were the night before.

One of the hardest things to do when grieving is to devote enough time to the work of grief. And it is work. Many employers only grant a few days off for grieving a family member, and this is woefully inadequate. As well, it can be hard holding down a full-time job while working through your grief.

The temptation is there to put it off, to throw yourself back into your life and avoid the uncomfortable feelings that grief brings. Elisabeth Kubler-Ross was one of the first researchers to take a serious look at grief when she studied the process among people with a terminal illness. In her legendary book On Death and Dying, she described **grief as a five-stage process: denial, anger, bargaining, depression, and acceptance** [11]. This process is not linear. We can find ourselves repeating stages, moving from one to the next and back again as our circumstances allow.

Kubler-Ross described the first stage as **denial and isolation**, which might mean asking for second opinions (or third, or fourth) from medical staff. It can be the way I felt disconnected from myself during the first few days after my boys died. It was as if the experience was happening to someone else. Pretending this is not really happening can be a way to shield yourself from painful emotions. It can be the way you simply do not want to go out, do not want to see others, and do not want to have to explain where your baby has gone.

The second stage is **anger**. This can be directed inward at yourself, or outward at others. You can even feel angry at your baby. You might be angry at the doctor for making a mistake, even if no mistakes were made. You might be angry at yourself for not recognizing "signs" your baby was in distress, even if those signs were all in your head. You can be angry at your partner, too, for not grieving in the same way you are, or for not being supportive enough of your concerns. You can be angry at other pregnant women for having healthy babies even though they do not deserve them.

The third stage is **bargaining**. This is where we try to take our loss and regain control over our world. We might make promises to ourselves or to God that this time will be different. "If I have a healthy baby, I promise I will ..." Often we do this sort of bargaining with ourselves to hide guilty feelings about things that happened in our last pregnancy. If you've felt guilty over the loss of your baby, it can be hard to let those feelings go. Forgiving yourself is an important step to feeling better.

The fourth stage, and for many of us the one that has the longest impact, is **depression**. Depression is more than sadness. It hurts. This is where you can't get out of bed, where you get little pleasure out of life. There is nothing that can be said or done to cheer you up. Depression has been described as a black dog that follows you around, as a cloud, or as a filter that leaves the whole world grey.

The final stage is **acceptance**. Acceptance is not the same thing as happiness. It is the point where you have incorporated the death of your baby into your life, where your baby becomes a part of you and who you are. Thinking about your baby will still be sad, but not painful in the same way that it was during the earlier stages.

New pain can bring up old grief. A friend once told me about how he had a hard time coping when his dog died. It left him with a deep and mystifying depression. As a church minister, he was used to being the one to hold it together at funerals. Usually, he was the one who was asked to step in and take charge, but here he was, almost paralyzed by depression for months by the death of a dog. It seemed far out of proportion to what was really going on. Finally, his wife helped him realize the obvious. He was not just grieving his dog. He was grieving all the other friends and family who had died. He had not allowed himself to grieve before because he was busy keeping busy. When his dog died, no one looked to him for answers. No one expected him to perform the funeral or to help wrap up the estate. Being free of expectations, he was free to grieve, and so he did. And it hurt.

If you're trying again and haven't felt like you've reached the acceptance phase, keep working on your grief. It can and will come back to you when you least expect it. Work with a grief counsellor (you can ask your doctor for a recommendation). Devote the time you need to doing grief work. You will see recurrences of grief throughout your life. We all do. It is part of the cycle of our lives. Grieving never completely goes away, but postponing the hard work and hard emotions of grief will only make things harder later on.

When trying again, it can be especially challenging if you get pregnant just 12 weeks after your loss. When this happens, it means your milestones in pregnancy will all occur at the same time. Your babies will have similar due dates. Events such as ultrasound scans and memorial dates will happen at around the same time. Many women report they find this difficult, especially as their due date approaches. Living where I do, the changes in seasons are often dramatic. I have a hard time emotionally as fall comes around and the weather starts changing. It reminds me too much of the weather when my twins died. I know I would have had a hard time had my later children been born at any time close to their dates, which I like to reserve for Nate and Sam. But regardless of what time of year you get pregnant, anniversaries and holidays are difficult.

Regina's Story

My name is Regina, and I lost my little boy five months ago. He was stillborn; my placenta was too small for the gestational age. I am currently pregnant with my little rainbow; I am eight weeks. I moved to Canada six years ago with my husband, Scott. He is Canadian, so we moved here to be closer to his family. I am from Peru. Jacob was our first son, and all my pregnancy with him seemed fine. Now, I am sometimes lonely, scared, and sad. I know things I wish I didn't. I have learned that pregnancy is something you can never take for granted. It is a gift.

Mothers and fathers are often on different pages when it comes to trying again after loss, too. Negotiating with your partner over when to try again can be challenging, as couples often have different struggles and different perspectives. If you had medical difficulties during your last pregnancy, your partner may want you to hold off on getting pregnant out of a desire to protect you, both physically and emotionally. On the other hand, men often experience greater anxiety the longer the interval is between your loss and your next pregnancy [12]. Regina mentioned that her husband, Scott, felt he wanted to try again right away: "From the very first night that they told us we lost Jacob, I said I'm not having another baby. That's it. Scott was like, we have to try again. From the very, very beginning he wanted to try again."

Whenever you decide you are ready, it is a deeply personal decision that only you and your partner can make together. As hard as it may be, don't let others pressure you one way or another. Having another baby in your arms will not stop you from grieving the one you lost. It is not the solution to ending your sadness. You will continue to mourn your baby whether you are pregnant or not, so taking time to make your decision is perfectly okay. If you are feeling—either for medical or psychological reasons—that now is a good time, that's perfectly okay too. You can continue to grieve while pregnant!

Introducing Steph

My name is Steph, and my husband is Chris. I lost my son Liam at 39 weeks' gestation in 2011. I'm currently pregnant with our second rainbow baby; our first rainbow is nine months old. Her name is Grace. I'm not necessarily happy to be pregnant, I am more wary. When we began trying after my son, my first thought was how pregnancy had lost that "sparkle." That promise of new life and a new chapter. I'd been down that road only to be taken down a path no one thinks about until it happens to them. I talk about my son to anyone that will listen; sometimes it brings relief, sometimes waves of grief.

Steph and her husband talked about this when they decided to try again. She said, "How are we going to handle keeping his memory alive when we have another baby?" Unlike most of us, Steph was also able to get some perspective from someone close to her. Her own parents lost a baby before she was born. She describes a scene soon after her son Liam died: "My parents were staying with me to keep me company. When we were drinking coffee around the table, my dad was asking, 'What are you going to do? Are you going to have another baby?' And I said, 'Yeah, eventually.' And he said, 'I was just wondering, I think you should wait and save money.' And my mom got after him! She said, 'You can't tell them to wait! We didn't wait for a baby!' Two months later they started trying again and they had three losses before they had my brother. My Dad said, 'I'm just saying it was hard for us and I don't want her to go through that.'"

How Long Does It Take?

Once you decide it's time to start trying for another baby, you might be wondering how long it will take you to get pregnant again, especially if you had no trouble getting pregnant the last time or if your pregnancy was unplanned. The answer to that question varies widely and depends on several factors, such as your age, your partner's age, any health conditions you might have, and how well you are able to time having sex with ovulation. Some estimates show that in any given month, only one out of every five couples trying to get pregnant will be successful [13].

Another frequently cited explanation for how long it takes is that over the course of a year, 85 percent of couples who are trying to get pregnant will succeed. At some point, a well-meaning person has probably told you, "at least you know you can get pregnant," in response to your grief over losing your baby. As you probably know, that is not very helpful. Just because it was easy last time does not mean it will be easy this time. Another well-meaning person will also joke that "at least you can have fun trying!" Anyone who has struggled with fertility will tell you, there is nothing fun about sex on demand, for either you or your partner. Timing sex is frustrating and can lead to conflict in a lot of couples. Talk to each other a lot throughout this process to be sure you're on the same page.

There are natural family planning techniques you can use that might improve your chances. While natural family planning is not the most effective way to prevent pregnancy, knowing your body and your cycle can make getting pregnant a little easier. Start by keeping track of your menstrual cycles. This is probably something you're doing anyway. If your menstrual cycles are regular, every 28 or 29 days, this can be easy. Ovulation usually occurs sometime between day 10 and day 15, and most likely on day 14 or 15. You want to have sex every day or every other day during this fertile period. Sex after ovulation is not very effective. You can also use other natural family planning techniques, including tracking your cervical mucus or charting your basal temperature. These techniques are a little more complicated and involve monitoring your symptoms each day. If this is something you would like to try, a public health nurse or your doctor or midwife can teach you these methods.

Another recommendation is to avoid using lubricants, such as KY-Jelly or other brands, because this can affect sperm's ability to travel [14]. Avoid saliva. While the effect of saliva on sperm is small, it has some spermicidal quality. If there is a sperm issue affecting your ability to get pregnant, you'll want to avoid it.

If your partner smokes cigarettes or uses marijuana, both of these have an effect on sperm function too. Quitting or cutting back can help. It is hard to do, but can have big payoffs for both your health and his.

When Should I Seek Help Getting Pregnant?

As with the last question, the answer to this varies widely depending on both your and your partner's age and health. It also depends on where you live because the definition of infertile varies, and the point at which your health insurance will cover fertility treatment differs from plan to plan. Some jurisdictions will fund in vitro fertilization (IVF) treatment provided certain conditions are met, some jurisdictions will not. The technical definition of infertile is a couple who have not been able to get pregnant after one year of trying.

You should talk to your doctor if:

» you have been trying to get pregnant for more than one year
» you are over the age of 35 and have been trying to get pregnant for more than six months, or if your partner is over 50 [14]
» you have had more than one miscarriage
» you or your partner have known fertility issues (such as being a diabetic, having Polycystic Ovarian Syndrome or endometriosis)
» your periods are irregular

If you don't meet any of these criteria but are still distressed that you are not pregnant, it is best to see your doctor sooner. They can help you cope with the emotional roller coaster of trying to get pregnant.

Introducing Jenn

My name is Jenn, and I lost my baby girl, Fiona, just last year. She was full term and died during an induced labour due to complications with the cord and placenta. She was our miracle baby—our eighth attempt at IVF. We tried eight times over a four-year period. We went through three cycles and some frozen transfers as well, and none of them were successful, and nobody could tell us why. It was just a case of needing to keep trying, and so we did. We never thought it would work, and then to have it work twice in one year, it's just really unbelievable.

It was quite a journey to get pregnant in the first place, so I think our experience through our last pregnancy and this one are influenced by that struggle. With what happened to Fiona, we will be delivering this baby early, by a scheduled c-section. It was hard when Fiona died. I think people try to offer comfort by saying that we can get pregnant again and those sorts of things, but to us we didn't know. We don't know if it will be another four years and thousands upon thousands of dollars that we don't have. So there was no comfort for us in that, it's happened once it will happen again. We just really couldn't put any faith in that.

But from the other side of it, in those early weeks after Fiona had died, in a way Lucas [her husband] and I already had experienced all these losses along the way. We already had these established coping mechanisms for losing a baby, although it was just such a completely different experience to lose a child at full term compared to an embryo that didn't implant. But we'd been so used to everyone around us being pregnant and having babies and for years it seemed we watched as people joined this club that we could just not get membership to. In a way I think that might have made surviving a loss, like the one we had last year, a little easier, because we had all these ways of coping that we didn't even know we had.

All of Jenn's pregnancies were conceived through IVF, so she was already in the system when her daughter died. She knew as soon as she lost Fiona that she wanted to try again, even though they only had one frozen embryo left. She said, "It was almost a need, it was this most desperate need. Even in the hospital, Lucas and I talked about it. We had this one little frozen embryo left and we'd always imagined going back for it, you know, maybe in a couple years' time, just thinking the pressure would be off. And thankfully for both me and Lucas there was just this need to do that because I think if we'd been in different places as far as that was concerned, it would have been really difficult."

Alternative or Complementary Medicine

Many people seek alternative or complementary medicine to improve their chances at fertility. Depending on your or your partner's medical condition, there may be something available to help. Unfortunately, according to Natural Medicines, an impartial evidence-based organization that evaluates alternative or complementary medicine, the treatments available for infertility have unclear or conflicting scientific evidence. Much of the next section is based on their findings. Their recommendations are divided into three groups: mental and spiritual therapies; herbs, vitamins, and supplements; and physical therapies.

Mental and Spiritual Therapies

Anyone who tells you that the reason you can't get pregnant is because you "need to relax" is essentially telling you that your mental state can influence your ability to get pregnant. It is a powerful idea. Personally, I found the suggestion that I "just relax" to be more frustrating than helpful. However, there is some limited evidence that mental and spiritual therapy may have some benefit. Keep in mind, the key word in this phrase is limited. None of these therapies have very strong evidence of benefit. One suggestion is hypnosis. According to Natural Medicines, "based on early evidence, hypnosis may improve the in vitro fertilization–embryo transfer cycle. Additional study is needed before a firm conclusion can be drawn" [15, 16].

If you consider yourself a spiritual or religious person, you may find prayer to be of benefit as well. This, too, is supported by weak evidence that it will help you get pregnant: "The potential effect of intercessory prayer on pregnancy rates in women being treated with in vitro fertilization–embryo transfer has been studied.

Preliminary results seem positive, but further research is necessary" (15). Prayer may help you feel better, feel more connected to God or your soul, or help you feel more connected to others. For these reasons alone you might find it worthwhile.

Finally, many health care professionals will recommend psychotherapy. Again, psychotherapy certainly can be of benefit in reducing anxiety or depression. It can help you and your partner feel more connected. However, there is limited evidence that psychotherapy improves fertility rates (15). If you are not yet seeing a psychotherapist for your grief, this may be something you want to consider for your own benefit, but a therapist can't help you get pregnant faster (17). With each of these mental and spiritual therapies, there is likely no harm, so if it helps you, go ahead!

Herbs, Vitamins, and Supplements

If you are interested in trying herbal medicine, vitamins, or supplements, there are a lot of options available. Unfortunately, there is little research demonstrating the benefit of these options. The research that does exist is often of poor quality. However, this does not mean you need to dismiss complementary medicine outright. There may be some benefits to these medicines. What follows are some of the commonly used supplements for improving fertility in both men and women, and what current research says about their effectiveness. There may be additional choices depending on your specific diagnosis. As with all medications, check with your doctor or pharmacist to be certain there aren't any unwanted interactions between these and other medications you might be taking.

If you aren't already, it is time to start taking a folic acid supplement or a prenatal vitamin. You can ask your doctor or pharmacist for suggestions. This may be of particular importance if you have celiac disease or a gluten intolerance. In many countries, including the United States, Canada, and Australia, folate or folic acid are added to grain products to ensure women get enough folic acid in their diet. At the time of writing this, the United Kingdom, European Union countries, and New Zealand do not. If you're not consuming grain products, you may be at risk of not getting enough. Low levels of folic acid are associated with higher rates of spina bifida, among other congenital issues. Take a look at the table on page 17 to find other sources of folic acid (18).

Other great sources of folic acid (based on a standard serving size)

Excellent sources (55 μG micrograms or more)

» cooked beans (face, kidney, pinto, roman, soy, and white), chickpeas, lentils

» cooked spinach, asparagus

» romaine lettuce

» orange juice, canned pineapple juice

» sunflower seeds

Good sources (35–55 μG)

» cooked lima beans, corn, brussels sprouts, broccoli, green peas, beets

» bean sprouts

» oranges

» honeydew melon

» raspberries, blackberries

» avocado

» roasted peanuts

» wheat germ

Other sources (11–33 μG)

» cooked carrots, beet greens, sweet potato, snow peas, summer and winter squash, rutabaga, cabbage, green beans

» cashews, walnuts

» eggs

» strawberries, banana, grapefruit, cantaloupe

» pork, kidney

» breakfast cereals

» milk

Supplements to Improve Male Fertility

For improving male fertility, some of the suggested supplements include astaxanthin, coenzyme Q10, l-carnitine, lycopene, maca, selenium, tribulus, and zinc. These are believed to either increase sperm count or sperm quality. Astaxanthin is a carotenoid, and is what gives lobster, salmon, and other seafood creatures their red colour. Although you can buy it as a supplement, the FDA does not allow it to be used as a dye in foods intended for human consumption. According to Natural Standard, "there is currently insufficient available evidence to recommend for or against the use of astaxanthin for male fertility. Additional study is needed in this area" [15].

Coenzyme Q10 is another supplement you may have seen advertised for a variety of conditions, including the suggestion that it improves sperm motility (how fast they wiggle) and sperm count. As with astaxanthin, "better studies are needed before a strong recommendation can be made" [15]. This is consistent with a Cochrane review on antioxidants for male fertility, which found only a small increase in the birth rate for men undergoing fertility treatment while taking supplements such as coenzyme Q10 [19].

L-carnitine is another supplement advertised as beneficial to sperm motility, although it is usually marketed as an amino acid designed to help bodybuilders build muscle. As with the other supplements, research is limited and there is not enough to recommend it [15]. Cochrane Reviews also looked at l-carnitine and found there was not enough evidence to recommend it as a fertility supplement [19].

Like astaxanthin, lycopene is another carotenoid. In this instance it is what gives tomatoes their colour. It too is said to improve male fertility, yet research remains preliminary. Maca is a plant native to Peru, and is believed to have aphrodisiac qualities and to improve semen quality. It has been used in Peru on both humans and animals to improve libido. It is also a root vegetable and can be eaten in a variety of forms. Eat it if you think it tastes good, but for now, there is not enough research to recommend it for fertility purposes [15].

Selenium is a common element that can be found in many daily vitamins for men and is believed to play a role in male fertility. At this stage, results are mixed. Some report an improvement in fertility [20]. Others are not conclusive [21].

Tribulus terrestris is another plant often used in traditional Chinese medicine as well as Indian Ayurvedic medicine. It goes by a lot of other names depending on which tradition you come from and whether you view the plant as a potential medicine or simply a noxious weed. Bodybuilders use tribulus supplements because they believe it increases testosterone levels. Early research on this plant seems to be encouraging. It appears to improve sperm motility and health as well as increase libido. Unfortunately, the research studies are of poor quality, so there is not enough to recommend this supplement (15).

Lastly, zinc supplements are often advertised as improving male fertility, by improving both sperm quality and sperm number. However, other research studies found it increased the number of abnormal sperm, possibly cancelling out any benefit. Because of this, the research remains inconclusive (15).

Supplements to Improve Female Fertility

Supplements for improving female fertility are believed to increase follicle stimulating hormone or regulate menstrual cycles. Some of the supplements suggested are dehydroepiandrosterone (DHEA), dogwood, green tea, and tribulus. As is the case with the male fertility options, for each of these supplements, the research is very preliminary and often of poor quality. A Cochrane review was also done on antioxidant use for female infertility, and like the male study, it found that most of the trials were of poor quality. As a result, there is not enough evidence to recommend antioxidants as a treatment (22).

DHEA is a supplement advertised to women for building muscle strength and fighting the effects of aging. There is some suggestion that "DHEA supplementation may be beneficial in women with ovulation disorders. There is currently not enough scientific evidence to form a clear conclusion"(15). Dogwood is used by practitioners of traditional Chinese medicine because it is believed to help improve levels of follicle stimulating hormone and luteinizing hormone. The Natural Standard review found only one study on the use of dogwood, so this is insufficient to make a recommendation (15). Green tea is another product that some early research indicates may be helpful, however "further well-designed research on green tea alone for this use is needed before a conclusion can be drawn" (15). The Cochrane review found only one study on green tea. In this study, it was blended with other products, so a comparison could not be made (22, 23).

Physical Therapies

If you're having fertility treatments, signing up for more needles is quite possibly the last thing you want to do. But acupuncture is a commonly used complementary treatment for improving fertility. So far there is only "inconclusive evidence in support of acupuncture for infertility" (15). A recent Cochrane review looking specifically at treating polycystic ovarian syndrome (a common cause of low fertility) with acupuncture found that there just wasn't enough evidence to recommend it (24). Acupuncture may benefit in the same way as mental and spiritual therapies. It gives you a sense of calm and control over your body and reduces stress. As with the mental and spiritual therapies, for many of the physical therapies there is likely to be no harm in trying them.

Exercise is a form of physical therapy and there are many options for becoming more physically fit. You would think there would be a lot of research demonstrating that exercising more and becoming more active would improve your fertility. But even in this instance, a Cochrane review on specific lifestyle interventions (things like diet and exercise) found there was not enough to suggest an improvement in fertility (25). However, their review only looked at people who were undergoing fertility treatment, not the general population. For both men and women, moderate exercise appears to be best for improving fertility (26). There is not enough evidence to recommend a specific type of exercise, from yoga to walking to swimming, so choose whichever works best for you (27).

This can be frustrating, as I found I struggled a lot with body image issues after losing my twins. I hated my body. I blamed it for causing my sons to die. If you had body image concerns even before your loss, losing your baby can amplify these feelings. While exercise may not be the path to a baby, moderate exercise can help you feel better about yourself. I found walking was a great way to work out my grief, so I would walk around my neighbourhood for hours, working out all that was on my mind. The last thing I wanted to do was see other people, so a gym or exercise class would not have worked for me. I know others who have tried yoga, and who find attending a class at a set time each week helps keep them motivated. Some people find exercise works best when they work it into their daily routine, such as riding a bicycle to work. Regina says, "When I lost him (Jacob), I went crazy at the gym. And it was for me— like— putting my music on my iPod and using the treadmill—all that anger that I had inside. It was like I went crazy. I don't know—it was for me a way of getting rid of all that anger that I had." Losing a baby and trying to conceive can make you feel out of control—of your own life and your own body. Exercise can be a healthy way to return to a feeling of control.

If you are hoping to do more than just moderate exercise or if you are hoping to lose weight, talk to your doctor about your options. Not losing the weight gained during pregnancy and gaining too much weight during pregnancy are both associated with an increased risk of complications in your next pregnancy. Making lifestyle changes can be hard, and you will need a lot of support in the process. Small changes can still make a big difference.

The Zika Virus and Microcephaly

As I write this, fear about the Zika virus is very high, and for good reason. A lot remains unknown about the virus and the damage it causes to unborn babies. We know that it can cause birth defects in babies born to mothers who contract the virus while pregnant, in particular a condition called microcephaly. Microcephaly literally means small head, and it can cause a range of other health problems. Microcephaly can also be caused by infections from other viruses too, such as rubella, which is why getting the MMR or measles, mumps and rubella vaccine is important (28). We also know that the primary way that the Zika virus is spread is by being bitten by the Aedes aegypti mosquito. This type of mosquito also carries the dengue fever virus, among others. It is found in tropical parts of the world, such as South America, Africa, Southeast Asia, and the Caribbean. These mosquitoes are not found in Canada and the United Kingdom, nor are they found in most parts of the United States and Australia. However, the virus is also believed to be spread through sexual contact, so having sexual contact with someone who has travelled to these areas may also put you at risk. If you live or have to travel to an area where the Zika virus is found, take steps to avoid being bitten by mosquitoes, such as wearing long pants and long-sleeved shirts and using bug repellent with DEET, picaridin, IR3535, oil of lemon eucalyptus, or para-menthane-dioldeet (all active ingredients proven to be effective mosquito repellents). Because information about Zika is changing rapidly, your best source of information is your local public health agency, your doctor, or **www.cdc.gov/zika.**

Introducing Maeve

I am now 19 weeks pregnant with our rainbow baby after suffering the loss of our precious first-born son Cord at 35 weeks. He was born in January of this year. Perfect in every way, we lost him due to a placental abruption.

My husband and I have been on a very emotional, challenging journey this year. So blessed and happy to be pregnant again, but still grieving and lost over the death of our son. I found it particularly difficult early in the pregnancy while dealing with my hormones as well as the emotions that this new pregnancy stirred in me. Shock. Joy. Disbelief. Anxiety. Fear. Love! I expect my feelings may intensify again towards the 35-week mark, when I contend with the emotions from my previous loss.

I am 35 years old and I run a successful small business with my husband Gavin. We live in a semi-rural area of Australia, about half an hour from our nearest hospital. This time around we are "high risk," so not only is much of the innocence gone from this pregnancy but it is also a far more clinical, medical experience. The great thing about being self-employed is that I have flexibility with my work. But it also comes with a lot of responsibility and pressure, particularly when it comes to staff. It also means I sometimes have to put on a brave face despite my inner turmoil. This pregnancy we have really tried to take things slowly, to appreciate every precious moment. My whole world changed because of our son. My whole view of myself, others, life, my beliefs— everything. The dust is still settling. I'm not sure entirely who this new version of me is, but I know parts of me are stronger, braver, and fiercer. Other parts are more fragile, lost, tender, and mindful.

3

I'M PREGNANT
Now What

So, you've just found out you're pregnant: the little blue (or pink) line has confirmed it. Good news! Maeve described it as a great feeling. In her words, "it wasn't until I found out I was pregnant again that I realized what it really feels like to be happy. I had this euphoric feeling I hadn't felt in the six months since we'd lost Cord." Jenn, too, was very happy to find out she was pregnant. She says, "I think I just smiled for the first time in two and a half months. In that instant it was definitely a moment of surprise and joy and disbelief." At the same time, no one would be surprised if you do not feel like celebrating just yet. You are happy. This is what you have wanted for so long. And you are excited too. A voice in your head is telling you that this time, for sure, everything will turn out okay. Still, there is another little voice inside your head. One that cannot help but feel worried. What if the test is wrong? What if the pregnancy doesn't last? What if it happens again? And how will you survive the next 40 long weeks? Finding out you are pregnant again after a loss leads to mixed emotions. Memories of the last time you were pregnant. Excitement at the prospect of having another baby. Fear that things will not work out. Sadness for the child you lost.

Over the next few months, you will probably feel the constant push and pull of not quite being fully engaged. One researcher describes it as having "one foot in and one foot out" of the pregnancy (29). As Jenn describes it, "we knew that the complications that led to Fiona's death were very unlikely to recur, so we didn't have that anxiety that the same sort of thing is likely to happen again. But I still worry that the baby's heart is going to stop beating, because I know it can happen." Because of this, you might be tempted to live in denial for a little while longer. By not thinking about this pregnancy, by not investing yourself too much emotionally, you think you are preparing yourself for the worst case scenario. However, even if you are not quite ready to post the good news all over social media, there are still a few things to take care of in these early pregnancy days. Start with yourself.

Choosing Your Practitioner

Some people have very little choice about who their medical practitioner will be. Maybe you live in a small town, and driving to a large academic medical centre would take too much time. Some of you cannot imagine changing providers at this point. That was how I felt. Despite how horrible it was to lose the boys, the fault did not lie with my doctor. I felt he was the only one who would be sympathetic to my experience. I just did not want to have to explain myself all over again. Some of you have no choice but to choose someone new. Maybe you have moved to a new city, or your doctor has since retired. If you are one of the many people who would like to find someone new to work with this time around, here are some tips on finding a new doctor or midwife.

First, remember that the doctor–patient relationship is just that: a relationship. There are some wonderful, kind, caring, knowledgeable providers who simply are not a good fit for your needs. This is not a reflection on either you or the practitioner's skills. It is simply a difference in personality. Like going on a first date, meeting with your practitioner is a chance to get to know them and determine if things will work out. They will not be offended if you choose someone else. Having this trust in someone new is especially difficult if you had a bad experience in the past. After her loss, Regina had to go to a clinic specializing in high-risk pregnancies that was over an hour away. The doctor had missed the diagnosis in her pregnancy with Jacob, so she was glad to be referred to the experts. Still, "it's hard, because I don't trust. I trust maybe 40 percent and then I can't. That's the sad thing. I know I should be trusting the doctors, but I don't. I honestly don't."

You might want to begin by asking your family doctor for a recommendation. Be open and honest about your fears. It is likely that your doctor may know by reputation another practitioner who will be able to meet your emotional needs or who specializes in caring for people with your medical condition. If you have had the same doctor for years, they should know you well and can help you find a good match. Asking friends and family may be helpful too, but chances are they have not experienced a loss like yours, so their needs may be very different.

If you are looking for an obstetrician, you can also go online. In the United States, you can get a list of obstetricians from the American College of Obstetricians and Gynecologists website. Other countries have their own physician directories that can help with this search. Unfortunately, there is often little information about their particular area of expertise, but unless you have had additional complications (for example, you are a cancer survivor), you will be looking for a maternal–fetal medicine expert.

Jenn found her doctor because she was the specialist who was on call the night her daughter died. She had never met her before but delivered very compassionate care at the time of Fiona's death.

Jenn describes it:

The night I was in labour, she was the one that told us Fiona had died. That's all kind of a blur to me now, but we saw her for a follow-up appointment to go through the post-mortem and at that point she said, "If you're going to try again, when it happens, get in touch with me and I'll look after you the best I can." We had the option of going to a different hospital, but because we felt so listened to at that appointment, it was so well done. She sat and cried with us. She was so honest with us, and gave so much in terms of support, in terms of acknowledging things that they didn't do right and really just explaining to us in a way that was really helpful to us. It was very sensitively and compassionately done.

Jenn phoned her just a couple weeks later and the obstetrical consultant brought her in for a scan the next week. During her pregnancy, the doctor has been very supportive, "not just in terms of frequent scans and lots of reassurance about the medical side of things, but the emotional support that I've had. Being able to go in there and cry and ask the most stupid questions and everything else. It is at the point where I'm now really anxious and worried about what I'm going to do without her, when everything goes according to plan and I don't have a reason to go back!"

You may be interested in choosing midwifery care instead. Midwives might be a better choice for you because they often have time for longer appointments. They often come to your home, rather than you having to go to a clinic. Midwives also deliver postpartum care. Current practice indicates that "midwife-led continuity of care confers important benefits and shows no adverse outcomes. However, due to the exclusion of women with significant maternal disease and substance abuse from some trials of women at mixed risk, **caution should be exercised in applying the findings of this review to women with substantial medical or obstetric complications**" (30). Many people who've experienced a stillbirth, early neonatal death, or multiple miscarriages are considered high risk, whether the cause was found or not. Depending on your circumstances, they may not accept you as a patient, but if this is something that interests you, it never hurts to ask. Even if you are not a good candidate for midwifery care, like your family doctor, a midwife will have insider knowledge about which obstetricians are good to work with and can make a recommendation. Choosing a midwife is a lot like choosing a doctor. In both instances you will want to ensure that your personalities work well together, and you can ask for recommendations from family and friends. In the United States, you can find a midwife through the American College of Nurse-Midwives, or through your state association.

Steph

Talks about her choices in finding a practitioner:

The first time, when I was pregnant with Liam, I went to midwives and I wanted to do the natural thing. One of the hospitals here had nurse-midwives, so they had a nursing background. If something did happen, then they knew how to handle it. And they were already there at the medical centre. When I got pregnant with Grace, they were very sweet. They said you can see us, but usually people that have a loss, they don't come back to us. They want to be monitored more closely. But it's up to you.

She talked with her doctor about it and felt she had good support there as well but was glad "it was our choice. The nurse-midwives at the hospital were totally okay with taking me as a patient." Still, not everything was the same, as the hospital had built a new wing in the interim between the loss of her son and her next pregnancy. So even though "it was in a different wing, all the nurses are familiar with me from last time. I felt like it was a good thing to move because I lost my son and I miss him like crazy, but I needed to focus on this baby, to keep her healthy and to keep myself healthy during the pregnancy. So I think it was a positive thing to move." Steph emphasizes how important the relationship between doctor and patient can be. As she says, "I've met other baby loss moms who don't have a good relationship with their doctors. Doctors that belittle their loss, or belittle their worries or their feelings about the pregnancy after a loss, and I really feel bad for them, because I didn't experience that."

Maeve had to make the switch from a midwife to an obstetrician because she is now considered a high-risk pregnancy. She says, "I have a very good obstetrician now. She was recommended to us from Karen (the midwife). And the only thing I'll miss with Karen is that advocacy role." She found it difficult when her obstetrician was on holidays because "they didn't want me to see the community midwife anymore because I'm high risk, so I had to travel to the hospital every time. It is painful, both emotionally because it's a huge trigger for me, and physically because of our work. I don't like to go up there by myself anymore so that means both Gavin and I have to take time off work to go to the hospital." Maeve continued to email her midwife for additional support and advice during the next pregnancy. Her first midwife was a specialized bereavement midwife.

When arranging for an appointment, let the administrative assistant know your medical history and ask for a slightly longer appointment time. This will both give the doctor or midwife the heads-up that you are not a typical patient, and ensure you have the time to have all your questions answered. Remember, this initial consultation is your chance to determine if you are a good fit, so do not be afraid to ask questions and do not be offended if things don't work out the first time. You may have to meet with a couple providers before you find one that is right for you.

Whichever type of practitioner you choose, knowing how decisions are made in health care can help you communicate with them. For over 20 years, health care practitioners have been following a model called evidence-based practice.

A common definition of evidence-based practice is the "conscientious, explicit, and judicious use of current best evidence in making decisions about the care of individual patients. The practice of evidence-based medicine means integrating individual clinical expertise with the best available external clinical evidence" (31). What this means is that the practitioner will take **three elements** and weigh them when making decisions.

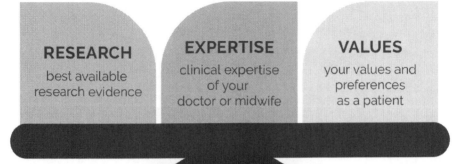

Fig 1: Evidence-Based Practice is the intersection of three components.

First, the best available **research evidence** related to your issue. Second, their own **clinical expertise**. Third, **your values and preferences** as the patient. When you meet with your practitioner, **they should be familiar with the latest research** and be willing to investigate answers to your questions, no matter how obscure. There has been very little research done on the experience of pregnancy after a loss, but they should be following the most recent practice guidelines.

The second element, **their experience as a practitioner**, is equally important. This is where their education and knowledge of local circumstances comes into play. These qualifications are particularly important when dealing with pregnancy after a loss, because of how little research is available on this subject. The practitioner will need to be willing to take that research and be able to share it with you in a way you can understand.

Finally the third element of health care decision-making is the **needs and desires of the individual patient**. Your practitioner should listen to your concerns, understand them, and work with you to find a solution. They should be able to explain their decision-making in a way you can understand and help put you at ease. If you feel your questions are dismissed, or if the practitioner is not explaining tests and procedures—and the risks and benefits of these procedures—in a way you can understand, then it is okay to walk away and find someone else.

Your practitioner should also be someone who works well with others. My physician was quick to refer me to a nurse practitioner and a social worker for additional emotional support. If you have additional medical concerns, they may need to work with other specialists. Ask what other professionals they will be working with to ensure you get the care you need.

Choosing someone new or a new hospital is not without a downside. Regina had to go to a new hospital because her local hospital did not take high-risk patients. She described the new hospital as "strange. I had a friend, she had a terrible experience at [local hospital]. That's why she refuses to go back to that hospital. But in my case, the experience was really nice. I mean, it wasn't traumatic or anything. I don't feel like I don't want to be there, it's the opposite! I feel like I want to be there. I feel like I want to finish this. That I didn't finish the first time. I want to come back and I don't think I will feel like that if I go to [large hospital]." Because of the distance, she still needed to see her family doctor for some things, and was glad that she did. At the large hospital "I spend more time talking to the nurse and the technicians than with the doctor. I'm glad I have my doctor here for when I have concerns. I feel like I can talk to her, like she doesn't mind spending 30 or 40 minutes talking to me, where at [large hospital] I just feel like I'm rushed. But they do all the tests and stuff. That's the only reason that I go." When I talked to Regina toward the end of her pregnancy, she was glad to be going to the large hospital. She said "I feel a little bit of pressure from my family doctor here, regarding having the baby here. I feel that she wants to, that this is something she wants to see. And I feel like I'm in between, I don't want to hurt her feelings, but I can't risk anything. I don't want to risk anything more. I want to be safe and have the baby in [the large hospital]."

Telling Others

With the presence of social media, it is hard to avoid pregnancy announcements, and they seem to be getting earlier and earlier. Maybe those of us who have experienced a pregnancy loss notice them more. Whatever the case, you may be both reluctant to tell others the good news or eager to let them know. For some women, the thought of telling people right away was horrifying.

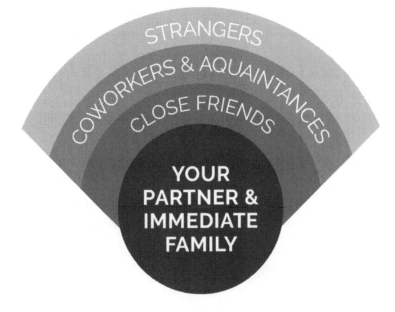

Fig 2: My personal circle of trust. I told different
people the good news at different times.

Certainly that was the case for me, as I already felt very much on display. Working mostly with women who knew my history of loss, I felt watched like a hawk. Telling them that I was pregnant at this early stage would have simply opened me up to more scrutiny that I did not need. I told my husband and that was it. Once I felt more comfortable, I posted to a listserv for women going through pregnancy after a loss. This was a huge support network for me—other women who knew that I was not completely crazy for feeling the way I did. Only after I heard a heartbeat did I tell other close family, like my parents and my sister. Next, and only after the 12-week scan, I told friends, including posting to Facebook. I never told anyone at work at all, but instead let them guess on their own. I knew that the law in my jurisdiction required me to give 30 days' notice before taking maternity leave, and I was pretty certain they could figure it out before then. It was also easy to hide my doctors' appointments, because my job involves meeting with a lot of doctors and no one would find it odd that I ran across the street to the hospital for a meeting with one of them. You might not be in the same position. Severe nausea and vomiting might make your pregnancy symptoms a little harder to hide, or you might need significant time off to attend appointments.

For many people, the first few weeks are a time to savour the news, just you and your partner. I began to think of who and when to tell as the different layers in a circle of concern. Where exactly people fit in this circle will depend on how close a relationship you have with them. How soon you tell people will depend both on where they fit in this circle and your own comfort level. It is up to you to gauge how much support you need from people in the circle and when to bring them in. Regina describes telling people about her new pregnancy: "Right away we told my mum. The first time, with Jacob, we told everyone. To me, waiting for the first three months was strange. Back home, we tell right away. This time it was different. Right away I told my mum and my mother-in-law, my sister-in-law. Then I was really, really picky about who I told or not. Because you find different reactions and some people think that they can judge, and I'm not willing to hear silly things. I decided who I say things to and who I don't."

Another person it can be hard to tell about the upcoming pregnancy are your living children, if you have any. If they are old enough to remember their sibling who died, you might find yourself having to manage their anxiety as well as your own. Maeve's two stepchildren were old enough to remember Cord's birth, and she described how difficult it was when the anniversary of his death came closer. "You know, he was actually excited about Cord's birthday. When I was sad the night before he was like, 'Yeah, but tomorrow is Cord's birthday. It is going to be great.' I said to him it is not quite the same as having him here. He sort of digested that a little bit and said, 'You can be happy about the next birthday you are having with this baby.' I thought I really have to hold it together for him. And we did." My daughter was not born when I lost my twins, and she was only two when we became pregnant again, so telling her about the upcoming baby was not as emotionally fraught. We chose not to have a discussion with her until I was very visibly pregnant.

4

YOUR EARLY PREGNANCY

The next few chapters are a week-by-week pregnancy guide that will take you through the common fears that come up during a pregnancy loss and the tests and procedures that might take place. There will be small insights as to what is going on with your baby, from when they first start to hear your voice, or what body parts are developing when. I begin with week five, not because there is nothing happening before that, but often because you only find out you are pregnant around week four. Dates in pregnancy measure from your last menstrual period, or LMP, so it is roughly two weeks before ovulation when pregnancy actually happens and another two weeks from ovulation until you can take a pregnancy test to find out if you are pregnant: the dreaded two-week wait! Whether you want to skip ahead and read it all the way through or work through this book one chapter at a time, as it coincides with your pregnancy, is up to you.

Week 5

This may be the first week you experience any real pregnancy symptoms other than a missed period. Chances are you are obsessing over every symptom. Nausea, fatigue, tender breasts, strong sense of smell: all of these you will interpret as a "good" sign. It means you are still pregnant! It means that things are happening normally. You may find yourself comparing these symptoms to ones you experienced during your last pregnancy. "I'm feeling way more nauseated this time, does this mean this pregnancy is stronger? Or does this mean something is wrong?" Or, "I'm nowhere near as exhausted as I was during my last pregnancy. This must be a bad sign." You can ruminate over each symptom endlessly. One suggestion is to write down your symptoms in a journal to record how you are feeling and to detect any patterns. This helps prompt your memory when you are at the doctor's office. It also makes it easier to put things out of your mind when you need to. Remember that every pregnancy, and every person, experiences different pregnancy symptoms. Work on managing the ones you have and not worrying about the ones you do not have. Journalling your symptoms and your feelings around them can help you feel a little more in control over your experience. Steph uses a blog and Pinterest as her journal. She describes it as very helpful: "If I don't write it down in the blog or on the computer, then I write it in a little journal, more to just get that weight (of anxiety) off. I've actually had people, because I put them on Pinterest, comment, 'I've clicked on this because of the picture and I didn't expect it to take me here. Thank you for sharing.' So it reaches people you never expected it to reach." Whether you make your journalling public or not is entirely up to you. Others have found writing letters to their unborn baby about their fears, their symptoms, or their lost child to be a therapeutic way to lessen anxiety.

Whether you are still happy living in denial or not, you will want to change your diet slightly starting this week. Some doctors will recommend cutting out some high-risk foods, such as fish with high levels of mercury (swordfish), unpasteurized milk products (such as soft cheeses) and processed meats which have a higher risk of listeria (such as cold cuts or hot dogs), and raw eggs, due to salmonella risk (goodbye Caesar salad). Listeria is very rare, so if you continue to eat these foods, be sure to pay attention to food recall warnings.

As difficult as it might be to avoid worrying, you do not need to obsess about your diet. One way to keep track of eating, especially if you are already using a journal to track your symptoms and emotions, is to keep a food diary. The Canada Food Guide has a simple downloadable guide with check boxes for each of the food groups. Every time you eat something, you simply check off the appropriate boxes. For me, because I love bacon, I used to have a bacon sandwich in the morning, with a chocolate milk. I would check off the boxes for dairy (one if I had a 250 mL size milk, two if I had a 500 mL size), for meat, and two grains (both slices of bread, or halves of the bagel). Because I am like most North American women, I found the fruit and veggie category lacking, so I began to adjust my diet and have fruit and yoghurt for breakfast instead. The visual cue reminded me of where I needed to focus my dietary needs.

Cat litter has been associated with toxoplasmosis, another disease that can be risky for your developing baby. If you have a cat, see if you can get your partner to clean out the litter box. If there is no one else to do it for you, use disposable gloves when cleaning out the litter box and be sure to wash your hands thoroughly. Also make certain it is cleaned frequently. Even if you do not have a cat, you should use gloves when gardening, because cats might be using your garden as their litter box.

Week 6

By week six, your baby is incredibly tiny: less than 0.01 inches (or two millimetres) long. Amazingly, this is the earliest possible detection of a heartbeat. Because I knew that, and because I knew that rates of miscarriage go down if a heartbeat is detected, I obsessed over getting confirmation of that heartbeat, especially after my first couple losses (32, 33). With my second pregnancy (first miscarriage), I did not even think about hearing a heartbeat, because I had no doubts everything would be fine. It was only at the ten-week mark that I began to bleed a little; an ultrasound was ordered, and no heartbeat was found. With my third and fourth pregnancies, I tried to stay in denial a little longer and not worry about hearing a heartbeat so soon. But with pregnancy five I was obsessed. I needed to hear that heartbeat in the worst way. My doctor arranged for an ultrasound at week seven, which he probably did because he wanted to balance my possible disappointment with reality.

Not being able to hear a heartbeat at week six truly is normal and not a sign that your pregnancy is doomed. Schedule the ultrasound too early and you will hear nothing, despite the fact that there is nothing to be concerned about. Schedule it later and you spend needless weeks fretting about whether the pregnancy is developing normally. In pregnancy five, the wait until week seven proved too much for my frantic mind. In the midst of a full blown panic attack, I took myself to the emergency room. The staff there were not impressed with me. I waited all night, abandoned in an examination room ("Our ultrasound machine is broken," is what they told me!), and found myself in the imaging department first thing in the morning. I got my ultrasound, heard my baby's heartbeat, and went home to rest at ease, knowing baby was okay. If they had not been able to detect anything, that would have been okay too, although I doubt I would have been able to convince myself of this. If you are the type who needs to know, ask your doctor what is the earliest she will schedule an ultrasound. Ask yourself, and her, about how best to manage your anxiety until then. It can be a long wait for some women, as higher body mass index can make it harder to hear the baby's heartbeat.

Week 7

What was smaller than a grain of rice last week has now changed to have a defined umbilical cord. And not much else. There still are not really any discernible body parts, other than maybe some little knobs that will eventually be the baby's arms. The head is starting to distinguish itself from the rest of the body but is not quite there yet. If you are going to experience morning sickness, it is around this time that you will first start feeling that awful rolling sensation, either first thing in the morning or all day long. Some women experience it even earlier, as soon as they are pregnant. About 75 percent of pregnant women report feeling nausea or vomiting. Fortunately, odds are you will not require hospitalization for your morning sickness. Only about one percent of women are hospitalized for hyperemesis gravidarum, which is the medical term for excessive vomiting during pregnancy [34]. With my first pregnancy, I cursed every time I vomited, which was about six times a day. I felt wretched. In fact, I gave my parents the wonderful news I was pregnant from the floor of the bathroom. My doctor prescribed Diclectin for me, and over time as I increased the dosage, I got to a point where at least I was not losing any more weight. And I mostly was not vomiting. I still felt horrible, but it was an improvement. There is some suggestion that morning sickness is correlated with a sensitivity to the pregnancy hormone hCG, so feeling sick is a sign the hormone is still present [35]. Keep in mind that there is a large range of normal hCG levels, and a large range of tolerances too, so just because you do not have morning sickness it does not mean there is a problem.

If you are feeling sick, you do not have to just suffer through it. In most countries, prescription medication is available to reduce the symptoms of hyperemesis gravidarum, which can be quite dangerous, as was the case with Katherine, the Duchess of Cambridge, and many other women. This is not the time to be losing weight, especially if you are thin to begin with. Severe nausea and vomiting are not just uncomfortable, but can cause you to shed pounds, putting you and your baby at risk. Ask your doctor about what your options are, and see if you can slowly increase the dosage of the medication until you find out what is right for you.

Over-the-counter medications and natural remedies can also help with your sickness. You can ask your doctor or pharmacist about these options too. Over-the-counter medications include Dramamine (dimenhydrinate). There is also some scientific evidence that acupressure, or shiatsu, can help relieve nausea and vomiting in pregnancy [36]. Pressure is applied on the P6 (or Neiguan) acupoint. You may see commercial products available that help to apply this pressure, such as Sea Bands. Ginger is another commonly used remedy for nausea and vomiting in pregnancy, although research has indicated it is only useful for a limited period (about five days). As with all medications, be certain to stay within the recommended dose, as some researchers warn against large doses of ginger due to associations with birth defects and miscarriage. Also, ginger is not recommended for use with blood thinners or with inflammatory bowel disease, and should be used cautiously with other conditions, such as diabetes. With any of these suggestions, either natural remedies or conventional medicine, you will want to talk them over with your health care practitioner. There may be specific reasons why your health care needs are unique and these products are not a good choice for you.

Better Living Through Chemistry?

Ingesting Chemicals

One of my first worries after discovering I was pregnant was about the chemicals my baby might be exposed to. At the time, the news was filled with stories about the chemical BPA (bisphenol A) in plastic water bottles. BPA is a chemical compound used in making plastics, and some research suggests that it can leach into our food, potentially causing problems, such as changes to the genital tract, to a developing fetus. I was lying awake at night worried about whether the BPA I had ingested would harm my child. Should I only drink tap water? On the other hand, tap water contains chlorine, among other chemicals. Would I ever safely drink water again?

Chemistry 101

Learning a little more about chemistry can help ease your anxiety. Chemistry was never my best subject in school, but here is my attempt at explaining why we need not fear chemicals—most of the time.

Chemicals are all around us, and they always have been. Chemicals are found in nature and can be classified in several ways. They can be organic or inorganic. They can be naturally occurring or man-made. What they cannot be is "good" or "bad." They do not have moral properties.

Organic and inorganic have different meanings when it comes to chemistry. While we may be used to the definition of organic produce as vegetables grown without pesticides, the term "organic" in chemistry simply relates to carbon. Organic chemicals are compounds that contain carbon, while inorganic chemicals do not. Petroleum is an example of a naturally occurring, organic compound. Table salt is an example of a naturally occurring, inorganic compound. Both can be harmful: petroleum in a small amount and table salt in a larger amount. The famous saying, "the poison is in the dose," means that whether something is harmful depends on how much of it you ingest.

Many chemicals that are perfectly safe can cause problems in specific situations. Aspirin, also known as acetylsalicylic acid or ASA, is a safe drug that is used to treat minor pain. Millions of people, including pregnant women, use it every day at safe doses, with no issues. However, a small number of people (less than 0.6 percent of the population) suffer from an allergy to this drug [37]. For them, even a regular dose can cause them to have a reaction, occasionally even anaphylaxis. And for all of us, taking too much Aspirin can cause death. Aspirin is not a bad chemical, just bad in particular situations. For pregnant women, a low dose Aspirin (81 mg) is safe. Consult your doctor or pharmacist before taking a higher dose. Another example is decongestants, which can raise your blood pressure. For people who already have high blood pressure, this can be a concern. For the rest of us, decongestants are just fine.

Finally, there are also drug interactions. These occur when two perfectly safe chemicals are taken together, but should not be. For example, grapefruit juice and a class of drugs called calcium channel blockers cause an interaction when they're combined. A chemical in grapefruit juice interferes with your body's ability to absorb the drug in calcium channel blockers, making them less effective. Again, neither of these chemicals are bad, but they should not be used together. Knowing this helped me put my fears about chemicals into perspective. And, even if some of your fears are a little irrational, if you have a history of loss, that is not a surprise. Be good to your body and yourself. Your pharmacist is a great person to ask for more information about particular medications in pregnancy. Here are some links to online sources too:

The US Government website **womenshealth.gov**. They have a great fact sheet that explains the different categories of medicine for pregnant women, from A to X.

The Organization of Teratology Information Specialists has both a website www.mothertobaby.org and a toll free number in the US to answer your questions about medications and both over-the-counter and illicit drugs in pregnancy. Their toll free number is **1-866-626-6847**.

Antidepressants in Pregnancy

One of the most common medications taken during pregnancy is antidepressants. An estimated 10 percent of women of childbearing age are taking antidepressants, and you might be concerned about whether you should continue to take them. That is a decision only you and your doctor can make together, as there are risks involved with quitting them, especially if you stop taking them abruptly. But what about the risks of continuing to take them? The research is not entirely clear. The largest and most recent review on the topic suggests that any risks taken are low [38]. In this review, the researchers looked at all the articles previously published on the topic. On three measures, the authors found a statistically significant difference. First, the babies were born on average three days earlier than the babies whose mothers did not take antidepressants. Second, the babies were born on average about 2.5 ounces (75 grams) lighter. Lastly, the babies had slightly lower Apgar scores at one and five minutes (half a point). However, the authors make clear that there might be other reasons for these differences, such as the presence of depression and stress contributing to lower birth weights or preterm birth. The authors did not find a link between antidepressants and miscarriage or stillbirth, although they also mentioned that only three studies were available on the topic of high enough quality to consider.

During my first pregnancy after loss I took Celexa. I was still very depressed and also nervous about quitting the medication altogether. With the guidance of my doctors, I weaned myself off the drug slowly, so I was not taking any by my third trimester. With my son, I was no longer taking antidepressants because I was in a much healthier place mentally. However, I did end up having to take much more powerful medications, including morphine, when I developed pneumonia. Whether you need to continue medications or would like to try to reduce or eliminate what you are taking, you can use the information sources mentioned above, and above all, talk with your doctor about your options and what the benefits and risks of each might be.

Week 8

What is going on in there? By this point, that little grain of rice has grown enough that the beginnings of arms and legs have formed, as well as eyes and the digestive system. This is about the earliest that the head and body are clearly identifiable on an ultrasound without magnification, so things are still pretty small (39). Despite their small size, the teeth, palate, eyes, and ears are all starting to form.

By this time, you have hopefully met with your doctor or midwife and are developing a great working relationship. Research into women who have had a pregnancy after a loss shows that they are often extra vigilant and cope with worry and anxiety by calling their care provider more frequently than women who have not had this experience (40). When you meet with your doctor or midwife, ask if email or telephone calls will be accepted, and what other ways they suggest for helping to manage anxiety. A lot of women also try to downplay their fears when they meet with their care provider. You have no need to do that. Any obstetrician or midwife should be aware of how your past history is affecting you and should recognize that your concerns are valid.

Seeing your care provider more frequently can be challenging, especially if you have to travel a long distance or do not have a job that is flexible. Just going back to the same place your child died can be a trigger. Steph talks about the ritual she has that makes it easier on her emotionally: "I have this thing that I have done as I go from my office to the doctor's office. I take the main road through the main part of the medical centre and you pass all the different hospitals. I pass the entrance that we take, that we took to have Liam that day, and every time we pass it, I have his little picture, one of his pictures, hanging from my rear view mirror. Every time I pass it I rub it. So when I go twice a month, that's just something."

You might also want to ask about support groups for women experiencing pregnancy after a loss. Because women who are pregnant after a loss often feel as though they do not fit in with other mothering groups, a support group specifically for women like you may be a great help. In my smaller town, no such group existed, so while there were support groups for women who had lost a child, I did not feel comfortable going to them once I was pregnant. There were too many other women who were either still trying to get pregnant or unable to get pregnant. My pregnancy, and the hopes and dreams I had for my new baby, no longer fit with these women. I was afraid I was rubbing their faces in it.

On the other hand, traditional prenatal classes were a poor fit too. Meeting with women who knew nothing of loss, who were still naive and joyful about pregnancy, meant there was little understanding of how my fears and anxieties were important and valid. Certainly research has shown that support groups specifically for women who are pregnant after a loss are beneficial, and that weekly meetings can help reduce some of the stress and anxiety (41). If there is no in-person support group in your community, online support groups exist. These can be done through Facebook, listservs, or other social networks. They have the benefit of being available 24 hours a day, seven days a week, of being available even in rural and remote communities, and not being limited by size. Steph has used Facebook during her pregnancies for emotional support. As she says, "I'll go back to the little forums on Facebook and talk to other people, post my opinion if somebody posts something. I'll comment on it or something, help people that are newer in this journey than myself because I know that's how I felt when I first found them. That helped me a lot, knowing that I wasn't alone and knowing that there is light at the end of the tunnel. You don't have to give in to the depression, you don't have to give in to the grief." A downside of Facebook and other online informal groups is that they might not led by professional therapists or facilitators, so there may be little additional help if it is needed, or if the conversation gets out of hand. If in-person support groups work for you, your obstetrician or midwife should be aware of them and will be able to help you make the connection.

5

WEEKS 9-13

Week 9: Baby's Heartbeat

While you may have caught a glimpse of the baby's heartbeat on an earlier ultrasound, nine weeks' gestation is the point in your pregnancy where you can likely hear a heartbeat using a handheld Doppler. However, this is only true for women who are thin. If you were overweight or obese before getting pregnant, it can be harder to pick up the heartbeat sounds. In that case, you might have to wait another month or so before a heartbeat can be heard. A handheld Doppler, or Doptone, is the kind of small machine that you might commonly see in your family doctor or midwife's office, as opposed to the larger ultrasound more often used in obstetrical or fetal imaging departments. While the larger machine translates the sound into an image, either two-dimensional or three-dimensional, the Doppler only amplifies the sound, allowing you to hear the baby's heartbeat (42). Dopplers are relatively inexpensive (especially in the world of medical technology), relatively easy to use (again, compared to some complex machines), and generally considered safe. There are several brands of home Doppler units on the market, and even some more expensive professional models can be rented. Which leads to the question: is a home Doppler a good idea? The answer may not be straightforward.

There certainly are some benefits:

» No need to go to the hospital every time you suspect something is wrong.

» You can listen to baby any time you want.

» Your partner can listen to baby any time he wants.

Now for the downsides:

» If you cannot hear the baby's heartbeat, you will panic, sometimes with no cause for alarm.

» They cost money (especially the really good ones).

» It might not work well (especially if you're overweight).

» You just hear the heartbeat. Using an ultrasound, doctors can look at other factors to help them determine if baby's okay, such as the fetal movements, breathing movements, amniotic fluid levels, and blood flow. Hearing the heartbeat can give you a false sense of security.

» There may be some risk of harm to the baby.

Keep in mind, that the last point is based on the best guess of doctors, not on actual hard evidence, and even then, only in the first trimester. In fact, here is the direct quote from the International Society of Ultrasound in Obstetrics and Gynecology: "The main reason for advocating precautionary use of Doppler ultrasound in early gestation is not because we know that it causes harm, but because we don't know that it is safe, and because the first trimester is a particularly vulnerable period of fetal life" (43). Theoretically, because ultrasounds generate heat, holding the machine on one fetal structure for a long time might impact the developing baby. There are no studies of Dopplers used at home, which are nowhere near as powerful as the ones used in the fetal assessment units of hospitals and are considered safe to use by the FDA. My own doctor suggested I not use one mostly due to the first point. He was afraid I would not be able to pick up the heartbeat and would therefore send myself into an unnecessary panic.

Regina got a Doppler so that she and Scott could listen to baby's heartbeat at home. She says, "I wasn't sure at the beginning because I was like, no I can manage, but we just purchased one because I am getting a little stressed and if I feel something weird I just want to be able to hear the heartbeat. [It is too far to go to hospital and] all they can do is use the Doppler and hear the heartbeat, so that's why we decided to purchase one, so we can actually do that. It will be helpful, I think."

Steph also got a Doppler. She says, "My doctor was afraid that it would do more harm than good if I couldn't find the heartbeat. I promised I would only use it if I don't feel the baby moving. Then I only use it to find the heartbeat. My husband always does it and I just lie there. I promise to use it for good, I won't use it for evil!" In the end, her doctor gave her a prescription for a Doppler and she ordered one through the organization Tiny Heartbeats. Her father, who also had a pregnancy loss, encouraged her to get one too, saying "'They have to have a belt or something that you could wear all the time so you can hear baby's heartbeat.' And I'm like, 'Dad they don't have those!'"

Maeve's response to her Doppler was very similar. She promised her doctor, "I'll get this Doppler and promise not to be too attached to it. But if it gets to two o'clock in the morning and I haven't felt movement, then that's a better thing." Meaning that it would be better to have that reassurance in the middle of the night than to lie awake feeling stressed and unable to sleep! Of course, hearing a heartbeat only confirms that the baby is still alive. If your baby hasn't moved for a long period of time, this could give you a false sense of reassurance. Going to get it checked out by a full ultrasound gives a better picture.

Whatever you decide, talk it over with your doctor or midwife. Depending on where you live, you may need a prescription to purchase one. If you decide to get a Doppler, try to only use it sparingly and have a plan in place for what you will do if you are unable to pick up the heartbeat. As someone who drove herself to the hospital in the middle of the night desperately needing to hear that heartbeat, I can certainly appreciate how comforting that whoomp, whoomp, whoomp sound can be. Regina likes being able to use it first thing in the morning, because "I feel weird in the morning, so we can use [the Doppler] right away and it's there and I can hear [the heartbeat] and get on with my day."

Week 10

At 10 weeks old, your baby is no longer an embryo and is now technically called a fetus. What's the difference? Very little. According to a leading obstetrical textbook, "The end of the embryonic period and the beginning of the fetal period is arbitrarily designated by most embryologists to begin eight weeks after fertilization—or 10 weeks after onset of last menses" (14). So celebrate this arbitrary milestone in any way you want. The difference is that in a fetus, all the cells that go on to develop the organs have been established, even if they are not yet fully formed. In an embryo, these cells are still dividing (42).

At 10 weeks, your baby is about 2.5 inches (six centimetres) long (44). His or her eyelids are now fused shut—they won't open until much closer to your delivery date. The parts that will make up the intestines are migrating from the umbilical cord to inside the body around this time too. Other changes that happen around this week? If your baby is a boy, he'll begin producing his own testosterone. Your baby is also starting to produce digestive juices in his stomach and the beginnings of teeth buds.

Non-Invasive Prenatal Testing

Since my last pregnancy, a new test—non-invasive prenatal test (NIPT)—has become available. It is a simple blood test that can check for chromosomal changes, and is often done at around week nine or 10 of your pregnancy. Because some of your baby's DNA (cell-free fetal DNA) is found in your blood, the lab can look at the baby's DNA in your blood sample. The test looks for Down syndrome, sometimes called trisomy 21, as well as two other rare chromosomal diseases, trisomy 13 and trisomy 18 (also called Edwards syndrome). Non-invasive prenatal test can also identify the sex of your baby. The test is very effective for screening for Down syndrome, although if your test is positive and you are considered a high risk for having a child with Down syndrome, there will be further testing done to confirm this, such as chorionic villus sampling or amniocentesis.

Chorionic Villus Sampling

If your doctor recommends chorionic villus sampling, this procedure that will happen sometime between the 10th and the 12th week of pregnancy. Chorionic villus sampling (CVS) is a method of obtaining a sample of cells from the placenta, called chorionic villi, so that genetic testing can be performed [18]. This is usually done by inserting a needle through the abdomen, similar to the procedure in amniocentesis. Another method involves going through the cervix using very long and thin biopsy forceps. In both cases, the doctor performing the procedure will use an ultrasound machine to guide them and to be sure they are getting the sample correctly. There is an increased risk of miscarriage (roughly one in 100). The tests can help to predict over 200 possible genetic disorders. One advantage of CVS over amniocentesis is that it can be done a few weeks sooner, so you will get your results a little faster [45].

As with a lot of procedures, your past loss means you are likely to be much more anxious. That is especially true if your previous loss was due to a genetic condition. With CVS, you will want to relax as much as possible, both before and after the procedure. Consider creating a list of things you can do that help you relax, whether it is contacting your online support groups, reading trashy novels, or watching movies. In the immediate aftermath of the procedure, you will want to lie down or rest, so try to include some non-active options. Test results can take between one and two weeks to arrive, depending on your location and what conditions they are testing for, so you will need to ensure your stress-reduction plan will help you over the days to come. Below you'll find that I have purposely separated information/suggestions about what to do when things go wrong. The intention of this book is not to sugar-coat things. It was important for me to include them here, but if this increases your anxiety, go ahead and put this book down for a few days until you feel ready to come back, or just skip those sections altogether.

When It Happens Again

I wish I could tell you that once you have lost once, you will never have to face another loss again. We both know that is not true. I did not have a successful pregnancy until my fourth one, so both my second and third pregnancies after the stillbirth were miscarriages. It is horrible. There are no other words to describe it.

In both my second and third pregnancies, I had a blighted ovum. This is not actually a medical term. Essentially, sperm met egg and nothing happened. No baby ever developed. So while my body thought and acted as though it was pregnant, all this time there was never anything there. I took comfort in that thought, because in my mind it meant I did not lose another one. It was just my body playing tricks on me. Some women disagree and feel upset when the doctor tells them they did not really lose a baby, that there was never one there to begin with. The emotional pain of losing your hopes and dreams, especially for the second or third time, is still painful either way.

If you are facing another pregnancy loss, you will find yourself both grieving this loss as well as feeling renewed grief over your previous losses. It can be overwhelming. It can be additionally traumatizing if medical professionals are not caring and compassionate. Miscarriage is one of the most common reasons for emergency room visits (roughly one in 100 ER visits in the US are for miscarriage or threatened miscarriage) (46). It is also challenging for doctors and nurses because they feel powerless—there is nothing they can do to stop it from happening.

Just as there is not a right or wrong way to grieve a late stillbirth, there is not a right or wrong way to grieve a miscarriage. If you have taken steps to protect yourself emotionally, you may find you are surprised by the intense feelings of grief. On the other hand, you may also surprise yourself by not feeling much grief at all. Never let anyone else tell you how to feel, and take your own time in coming to terms with this loss as well.

I could promise you that next time will be different, but that would be a lie too. None of us can predict the future, although statistically most women who have multiple miscarriages eventually go on to have a child, as I did. Only about one percent of couples are found to have recurrent miscarriage (sometimes called by the awful term "habitual aborter"), which refers to women who have had three or more miscarriages in a row [47].

If you think you deserve better care, such as a more thorough evaluation of causes of miscarriage or better follow-up from your doctor, speak up. While there may be little doctors can do to stop a miscarriage, and 50 percent of miscarriages have no known cause, that is no excuse for poor treatment. Let the doctor know that supportive care for miscarriage exists and that you would find it helpful. This can include genetic counselling, psychotherapy, bereavement support, or hormonal monitoring in your next pregnancy [48, 49].

One of the women I interviewed ended up having another miscarriage, and it would be her last pregnancy. For Kim and her husband Owen, their son Eric was stillborn in 2008, and they already had a daughter, Emily. After struggling with fertility issues, her pregnancy after a loss was not planned. In her words, "We didn't have any inkling that anything like this would ever happen to us. It took us three and a half years to have Emily with rigorous, scheduled trying. After Emily was born I thought, okay, I'm 42, we are lucky to have a living child and we talked about whether we should have another one. I thought, I don't want to go through all of the charting and all of the temperatures and all that. I don't want to do it. So we weren't keeping track of everything. I didn't think it was going to happen. I didn't really make plans for this." She describes all of the things she tried to get pregnant with Emily and how stressful it was, things they didn't have to do when they became pregnant with Eric. "We sought IVF treatment with donor eggs. We tried acupuncture. We tried vitamins. We tried chiropractic. I gave up gluten. We just tried so many things." When she lost this pregnancy, finding out during an ultrasound at eight weeks, she realized that this would be her last. But it was still a big setback emotionally. She said, "sometimes

I find myself saying I am fine, coping with this fine. Then the next day or the next week I am a complete wreck." On the one hand, she was philosophical about her loss, saying, "We have to have death to make life important. You have to have bad things in your life in order to appreciate the good." On the other hand, it was frustrating to be told to feel grateful for her one living child. "I know all about being grateful and I know all about appreciating what I have. Don't tell me that I should be grateful. Why should I have to be the one who doesn't get to ask for more?"

When I found out I was pregnant with my daughter Rebecca, it was at a fertility clinic where we had gone for a consult. I did not realize I was already pregnant. However, there in the waiting room was an old friend I had not seen since we were in school together. I was not really sure of the etiquette, so I pretended I did not see her, then sent her a quick email as soon as I got back to my desk. I apologized for not saying hello, but that I did not think it was the right time or place and thought she might feel awkward. We rekindled our friendship immediately, although it was short-lived. We were on different paths. That same day in the doctor's office, I was finding out I was pregnant again. She was being told by the doctor that he did not think it was ethical for him to continue to take her money. After spending more than $70,000 on fertility treatments, the chances of success were just too low. It was time for her to call it quits. About three months after reconnecting, just as my pregnancy was starting to become common knowledge, she sent me a very nice note, letting me know that it was too painful for her right now and that she wished me all the best. I admire her so much for her honesty.

Whether we end up having living children or not, how do we know when to call it quits? For many of us who have lost children, it seems the answer is always "just one more." Just one more child and my family will be complete. Just one more try and this time, this time for sure I'll get pregnant.

I have two living children, but my family will never be complete. So many circumstances are beyond my control. I am sad about it, but I am comfortable with the sadness. I do not know for certain, but I imagine the process takes much longer when you have no living children. It does not help when the messages we receive from our culture are that fertility treatments are a cure-all and that success is guaranteed. Incredibly, even surveys of female medical professionals showed that they overestimated how easy it would be to get pregnant (50). Most people assume that childless couples are childless by choice, even if that is false.

If you have had another loss and are thinking about calling it quits, make certain it is a decision you are comfortable with. There is support available, and your doctor should be able to refer you to counselling. There is also a multitude of support groups online, such as **Childless Not By Choice** or **Life Without Baby**.

Week 11

Week 11 brings a few more small changes to your baby. Around this time, the webbing between the fingers and toes disappears (51). It is also around this week that you might notice you are starting to show. This can bring a lot of anxiety for women who have lost a pregnancy, because it means it is getting harder and harder to deny to others that you are pregnant. You might not be ready to be "out." It is not unusual to show a lot earlier in this pregnancy if you have had a pregnancy or two before. Your body is used to being pregnant and adjusts more easily to the changing hormones and changing shape pregnancy brings.

If you are feeling anxious that people can tell, you can probably relax. Few people would be able to notice the subtle changes in your body that are taking place right now. And even if they can, even fewer people would be bold enough to say something. You can probably keep things under wraps for a couple more weeks, at least. Baggy t-shirts and sweaters, flowing dresses and cardigans can all keep the gossipers at bay for a little while. Keep in mind, ultimately, that you can wait to tell everyone for a lot longer. Where I live, the law about maternity leave only requires me to give my boss 30 days' notice. While the law may be different where you live, that's quite a long way from 11 weeks pregnant!

Nuchal Translucency Scan

The nuchal translucency scan is often referred to as the 12-week scan because it is done roughly around this time, sometime between weeks 11 and 14 (18). For moms-to-be who have not had a loss, this scan is considered exciting as it is usually the first chance they have to see their baby, or babies, and it is sometimes when they find out baby's sex. However, scanning for sex is not very reliable this early in the pregnancy, so do not be surprised if you have to wait a little longer to find out if you are having a boy or a girl.

Only ultrasound departments that have been accredited by the Fetal Medicine Foundation can perform the nuchal translucency scan, so it will likely be done in a larger clinic or hospital. You may find yourself in the waiting room with other mothers who are very excited to be there, often bringing whole families to the "event." I spent the whole time wondering how they would react with all those other people in the room if they got bad news. The nuchal translucency scan is done to test for Down syndrome by measuring the amount of fluid at the back of the baby's neck. In the case of babies with Down syndrome, there is more fluid than normal. This test is done at the same time as the blood test called maternal serum screening, and the results are read together. The test is not conclusive, so if you test positive, you will likely have to undergo more testing, such as amniocentesis.

Many women who have had a loss report greater anxiety around ultrasounds, such as the nuchal translucency test, even if their loss was not related to this issue (52). It may be the first time you have to go back to the hospital where you received the bad news that your baby had died. Regina says, "With the scan, I just remember when my baby didn't have a heartbeat, so my first question is always, 'Is there a heartbeat?' And then, when I know that it's okay, you can continue." Steph felt much the same way. She talks about going to see her doctor and "she uses a Doppler and it takes her a lot to find the heartbeat. I'm just laying there and it feels like an eternity, but I don't want to worry her. I don't want her to know I'm worried sick yet, but it just feels like an eternity."

If this is the case for you, knowing that this is an event that can bring traumatic feelings helps you to be better prepared. While you might not want to bring in your entire family, it is okay to bring in support, either your partner or someone else. You can ask when booking your appointment if the ultrasound technician can be made aware of your past history. The technician can then try to accommodate you. Making sure you are the first appointment in the morning (less time spent in the waiting room), placing you in a different examination room than where you were when you received the news of your baby's death, and ensuring they listen for a fetal heartbeat first are some ways your worry might be eased.

Where to Turn If There Is a Problem

Genetic testing and first trimester screening are done to provide the best information possible to help guide your decision-making. In most cases, nothing is wrong. However, sometimes something is found on a test that means you have to make a decision. This could be the easiest or the hardest decision you have ever made. Decision-making around your prenatal results can be complicated if you have lost a baby before. You may be feeling renewed grief or guilt over decisions you made in your previous pregnancy. Those feelings are normal.

Whatever your diagnosis, genetic counsellors and your doctor should be there every step of the way. They should be the first people you talk to. They can help you find quality, reputable, current information about whatever diagnosis they have given you. Ultimately, when you talk to someone else who has been through what you've been through, you are still asking for their personal opinions about their personal journey. In truth, no one has ever stood in exactly the same position as you. Each of us has unique circumstances. If you choose to research online, don't just go to Google, but start with reputable sources, such as the National Library of Medicine's MedlinePlus or the **March of Dimes**. Your genetic counsellor or doctor can help with this too. Author Sherokee Ilse's new book, **The Prenatal Diagnosis Bombshell: Help and Hope After Continuing or Ending a Precious Pregnancy**, deals with coping after you have been given this challenging news. If you decide to terminate this pregnancy, **A Heartbreaking Choice** is a website with resources to support you through this decision. If you decide to continue with this pregnancy, ask your genetic counsellor to refer you to a support group related to the particular diagnosis you have received.

Week 12

At this point, your baby is starting to lose his or her tail (yes, babies have tails), and fingernails are beginning to grow. The bone marrow is starting to work to create blood. Whether the baby is a boy or a girl, the genitals are starting to develop, so it might be possible to determine gender on an ultrasound at this stage, if baby is positioned well and there is a clear view. As I mentioned earlier, it is still really early to make that distinction, so even professionals regularly get it wrong at this stage.

Coping with Disappointment over Sex or Number

While most people might say, "Just be happy you have a healthy baby," it is not unusual for women pregnant again after a loss to find themselves disappointed, either because the baby is a different sex from the one they lost, or because they are not expecting multiples. Both of these feelings are normal and not a sign that you are not going to love this baby or be a good mother. I experienced both of these feelings when I found out I was pregnant with a girl, and by finding out that she was all alone in there! Of course, the opposite is true as well, and for some women, finding out you are pregnant with a baby of a different gender will bring relief, especially in the rare case your last baby died of a medical condition that is linked to their gender.

Whatever your feelings, take the time to acknowledge them. You will come to love this baby too. Even if they had been the same gender, every child comes with their own personality, likes and dislikes, and sense of self. Regina talked about her husband, Scott, and his feelings on gender: "He's okay with the idea of having a girl. He says we'll be busy with girl things. In some ways, even if it is a boy, he's not Jacob. But we were ready for a boy." If you do not plan to have more children after this one, knowing you will never get to parent a girl, or never get to parent a boy, can be tough.

When Steph found out she was having another girl, she said, "I was going to feel really nervous if it was a boy. I'm still nervous, but it's just a little more reassuring that it's another girl. I'm relieved because there's not that unknown. Because of what happened with our son, we didn't know if it would happen again with another boy. But Grace (their first living child) is here, so we know that this time it's going to be okay again." Gender issues can be challenging because of other people's expectations, too. Steph continues: "I'm Hispanic and my family was saying, 'Are you going to try for a boy?' And I'm like, no, I'm done. I have a boy. I have my son and that's fine. It's kind of hurtful, but it's not their life. I have my son and if everything goes well this will probably be our last one because I'm just tired of being pregnant and I'm glad for my daughter and for my son and the time we did have with him. And hopefully we'll get the same opportunity with this baby."

Jenn, too, had strong feelings about gender, which were complicated by the fact that she and her husband initially thought they were going to have a boy. At one of their scans, "Lucas and I were pretty sure we saw some dangly bits, so we were sure it was a boy. And both of us were worried about how that would feel, if it was a boy, because we'd both pictured ourselves as being with this little girl. So we had this week, or two weeks, of thinking, 'Don't know if it's definite but we're pretty sure it's a boy.' And we really came round to the idea. We actually started to get quite excited and we talked about names and I had seen this little Superman sleep suit that we thought would be great. So it was really good for us to think it would be just amazing regardless. And then we found out the next week that it's a girl."

After having lost a boy, Charlotte described finding out she was having a girl as a positive sign. "Don't get me wrong, I would have been delighted if it was a boy as well, but for me it was setting up a new pathway to walk down, and something for me to focus on. It's a new dream, and you dare to start making plans and a new dream around a girl."

It is at the twelve-week scan that you usually find out if you are having twins or triplets and if you have lost twins or triplets, finding out there is only one in there can also be heartbreaking. For me, it was a reminder that I was permanently "out of the club." Mothers of multiples are treated as special in our culture. When you do not have any visible twins, there is not that acknowledgement. It hurts. You may feel some relief, because it means that many of the health complications that come with multiples are things you will not have to deal with. I will forever have a pang in my heart when I see twins, especially identical twin boys.

On the other hand, if you have just found out you are expecting twins and you lost a singleton, you might be feeling mixed emotions too. A pregnancy that was already complicated by a past loss now has another reason to be considered high risk. Multiples face a higher danger of stillbirth, higher rates of preterm birth, and higher rates of disability. You might be concerned about the financial pressures, or about your own health. These fears are real, and even if you are excited, it is okay to acknowledge that not everything is sunshine and roses in Twinville! As with disappointment about the baby's sex, take time to think about how you feel and recognize that this too is normal and healthy. You will adjust to the new realities of parenting two or more children and you will be able to manage your fears. If you were not already, you will likely have your medical care transferred to a high-risk obstetrical unit once you are pregnant with multiples. Make certain you have an obstetrician who acknowledges your fears and takes the extra time with you that you need.

Week 13

Many pregnancy guides will celebrate this milestone as being out of the "danger" zone. If your losses were later in pregnancy, you know this simply is not true. However, it is worthwhile to mark this moment all the same, because week 13 is when rates of miscarriage do drop. You have successfully made it to the end of the first trimester, and that is something to feel good about. Hopefully, around this time you will also start to feel a little better physically. Maybe a little less tired or a little less nauseated. If the physical symptoms of pregnancy have been a challenge, that, too, is something to celebrate.

If your symptoms have not been strong, that can also be a challenge, because it is still likely too early to feel movement. That can be hard. Regina describes it like this: "Now that I don't have the morning sickness, sometimes I just don't feel pregnant and I just panic. Every time I use the bathroom I check for blood or anything. Sometimes it is a little bit overwhelming, but I guess that's just the way it is. So far, they say everything is okay."

WEEKS 14-18

Week 14

Week 14 is officially the start of the second trimester. Nothing magical happens this week, except maybe the usual magic that happens when you are growing another person inside you. Your baby will start to grow hair. Not all babies are born with a lot of hair, but both hair on the head and hair on the body starts growing this week. The hair on the head may stay, but the body hair, also called lanugo, will mostly disappear by the time they are born. If your baby is born early or small for their gestational age, they may still have some of this hair at birth. Here is an interesting fact: you can grow this lanugo hair back if you become dangerously thin, either from a disease like anorexia nervosa or weight loss associated with cancer.

Maternity Clothes and Starting to Show

It is not unusual if you are starting to show this early in the pregnancy, especially if you were thin to begin with. Many women also report that they started to show a lot sooner with their second and subsequent pregnancies than they did with their first. Your body is just used to pregnancy. This can bring conflicting emotions. Regina described it this way: "It was shocking to see my belly there again. I do not know how to explain it. It's weird. When I'm taking a shower and I see my belly again, I just remember my last month when I was pregnant with my son. It just feels unreal, I do not know why, but it does. This time my belly is a little bit bigger than with Jacob when I was four months. My doctor said with a second pregnancy sometimes the belly is bigger, but in your case you had just four months in between, and you were 36 weeks, so this baby is just taking all the space that the other baby just left."

Maeve also felt very vulnerable when she started to show so early. She says, "As soon as I was pregnant, I popped. My boobs, my tummy as well. I looked like I was already six months. I was paranoid people would know I was pregnant right away. So I was wearing baggy clothes and just being protective. Gavin was genuinely happy and so was I, but I still did not want to tell anyone, not even my family, not even my parents. Not even my support group, my [loss] mother's support group."

Whatever the reason, from hormones to bloating to weight gain, you might feel a little apprehensive about showing again. If you are not quite ready to tell family, friends, or coworkers your news, having an obvious belly can be both physically and emotionally uncomfortable. Depending on the season, you might be able to hide under loose fitting sweaters or sundresses for a week or two longer, but around this time you will probably be having to think about maternity clothes. For women with a pregnancy after a loss, this can bring up some emotions. Some women find themselves going to the basement and bringing up the box of clothes they put away after their baby died. If they are pregnant around the same time of year or season, these clothes will likely be suitable, except they are a tangible reminder of your last pregnancy. Pulling out the box and seeing the same sweater you were wearing when you last felt your baby move, or the dress you wore to your baby's funeral, can be tough. It also means making an unspoken announcement to friends and family who last saw that sweater the first time around. Being ready for maternity clothes means being both physically and emotionally prepared for questions.

Of course, buying new maternity clothes can come with another host of emotions. Sadness that you will not be able to use the old clothes again. Frustration at having to spend more money on clothes you do not really want. And fear, always a little bit of fear. Even if it is a small one, buying new clothes represents an investment. An investment in time and money on this pregnancy. This may be especially hard for women who did not get to use a lot of their maternity clothes the last time. Of course, the flip side is also true. If your losses were all in the early stages of a pregnancy, there might be a little bit of joy that you have made it far enough to need maternity clothes.

There are lots of options for finding maternity clothes without breaking the bank. Wearing new clothes that are different from your last pregnancy will make it harder for someone to recognize that dress, but if going to a maternity shop fills you with dread, try a consignment shop. You get to spend less on clothes (smaller investment). Plus, you do not have to get a sales pitch from the store clerk trying to sign you up for their baby club! You can also try finding maternity clothes online and ordering that way, so they come to your door in a brown cardboard box and no one is the wiser! If you have told a trusted friend the news, they may be able to let you borrow some of their clothes. Getting maternity clothes second hand is often a good choice. A lot of women buy maternity clothes they wear only a few times and are looking to give them away.

Is This Your First?

When starting to show, you will also find yourself faced with the horrible question asked by well-meaning strangers: "Is this your first?" Ouch. The answer to this question is one of the most hotly talked about on baby loss blogs and online communities. If you have other living children, this is an easier question because you can answer honestly "no," and will not be afraid of the follow-up question, "How old are your other kids?" If you do not have any living children, the question can be a nightmare. If you answer "no," you might find yourself in a tight spot with a complete stranger, having to explain that while this is not your first pregnancy, you do not have a baby.

If you answer "yes," you might find yourself feeling guilty for denying the existence of your child, and then having to face other awkward follow-up questions and comments. I had one woman say: "Pregnancy's awful! Do you not wish you could have twins, so you could get the whole thing over with at once?" I just smiled and told her it was an interesting theory, but not very effective in practice.

Steph also talks about coping with the question. She says, "When I got pregnant with Grace all these people were asking, 'Is this your first baby?' and I think, I'm never going to see you again, do I really want to get into what happened with my son? Or do I just say yes and move on. But every time I said yes it would hurt a little bit and I would apologize to myself for saying that. But I feel like sharing him is special. If this is someone that I'm never going to see, they do not need to know. They do not deserve to know about him. But other people, like my boss and my coworkers who I've become close to, they know about it because I go to the doctor so often." She also talks about how she does not want to tell strangers because she does not want to be talked about as "that person." She says, "I'm that person! I'm that person that someone knows that's a friend of a friend that that happened to!"

Maeve also talked about being the topic of questions once people can see that you are pregnant. She says, "Before I could have avoided those questions, but not so much now. I am probably rude sometimes. Not rude, but I really do not engage people in pregnancy talk. I never engage people in pregnancy talk. I cut people's questions off pretty quickly. It is really bizarre to me, even people who know me ask all sorts of questions: 'Do you know what you are having?' 'Is it a boy or a girl?' 'Have you chosen a name?' 'When are you due?' 'Are you so excited?' 'It is always so exciting!' Are you nuts? I feel like a Scrooge. I feel like a really negative, nasty person."

Charlotte had another saying she heard a lot that made her angry: "When you are a mother." As she said, "The whole 'when you are a mother, then you will know.' Do I explain to people that I am already a mother, thanks very much? I've done the most difficult thing that you will ever have to do as a parent, saying goodbye to my child! You can't have your heart broken by the loss of your child and not be a mother!"

Week 15

At week 15, your baby is mostly busy with weight gain. For the next few weeks, most of the physical changes will be small ones, such as the ears moving up to the right position on the head, or the body growing to be more in proportion. But even though the changes are small, each passing week makes for big changes. Your emotions may still be on a roller coaster, but physically, pregnancy symptoms are likely as good as they are going to get. You still are not as big as a house, so moving around is easier and heartburn does not keep you up at night.

Amniocentesis

Amniocentesis is a test done during pregnancy primarily for three reasons: to test for genetic abnormalities, to remove amniotic fluid if you have too much (a condition called polyhydramnios), or to test your baby's lung development [53]. It is also rarely used to test for infection in the amniotic fluid. If you have opted for amniocentesis to test for genetic abnormalities, this will usually be done between the 15th and 20th week of pregnancy. In many places, the test is routine for women over 40, because at this point, the risk of having a baby with a genetic abnormality is higher than the risk of having a miscarriage from the amniocentesis. According to the Royal College of Obstetricians and Gynecologists, the risks of miscarriage from amniocentesis are roughly one in 100, although some newer research indicates it is actually much lower, more like one in 1600 [54]. You may also be advised to have amniocentesis if you had a blood test and it came back positive for a genetic condition, or if your previous loss was due to a genetic condition. If you have a family history of genetic abnormalities, you may also be advised to have amniocentesis.

Amniocentesis can be scary. It involves a really long needle and a really scary topic—the risk that your baby might not be okay. That's something no one wants to acknowledge, but because it is scary, it is normal to be nervous about having this test. Ask your health care provider for help in your decision-making about having this test and talk about its implications. While amniocentesis is a safe procedure, it is okay to let your doctor know if you have concerns. They need to recognize your concerns and work to help you feel more at ease if you decide to have the test. Many people are worried that it will hurt because the needle is so long. But because the needle is larger and skinnier than the one used to take blood, many people find it hurts less.

Here's what will happen during an amniocentesis. First, an ultrasound will be performed to determine where the baby is lying. You might be given something to numb your skin, either by rubbing a cream on your belly in the area where the needle will go, or by using a small needle on the skin with a local anesthetic. Using the ultrasound as a guide, the doctor will use a long, thin needle (about two to five inches or six to 10 centimetres) to remove a small amount of amniotic fluid (about four to six teaspoons or 20 to 30 millilitres) that will be sent to a lab for testing. If you are squeamish, this is the part to not watch. There is no need for the needle to touch your baby during this procedure, which is why the doctor will be watching on the ultrasound machine. Once the fluid is sent to the lab, it can take up to two weeks to get the results back if a full karyotype is done. You can find out more about the test and see an animated video, at medlineplus.gov.

Perhaps the only thing scarier at this time than an amniocentesis is the two-week wait to find out your results. Here are some things that moms who've had amniocentesis had to say about the procedure and about ways to reduce your pain and anxiety:

"It was absolutely fine. It did not hurt at all....They just scan you and put some gel on your tummy...and put a needle in. It wasn't sore at all, I mean, I thought, it was like, 'Ooh, this horse needle going in,' but it really wasn't sore at all, not for me anyway" (55).

"The doctor basically said to me, 'Hold my arm,' so I held his arm and he got out what appeared to be quite a large needle. And I have an absolute fear of needles and I was convinced I was going to pass out, although I was lying down, but he literally just put the needle into my stomach and pulled it out, and within, I mean, it literally was seconds. It did not hurt at all. It felt like mild period pain, I guess, as the needle went in" (55).

"Second time round, I found the amniocentesis, it was much more uncomfortable...because the baby was small and the way it was positioned, they had to take the fluid from much lower down, and I think I was more unwell second time round. And the whole process was just more, it was more uncomfortable physically and I was much more anxious about it" (55).

"So I felt that prick going in, although it wasn't painful, but I could feel, had the sensation. And then it moved in, and then it seemed to be moving through nothing. There was no resistance as she was continuing to push it. And then I could feel it on like a second layer of skin underneath, but this skin was much harder than the skin on the surface of the body. And she sort of pressed it and pressed it, and I could feel the pressure and feel the pressure, and then suddenly phut, it went through and it hurt a bit. And I jumped—which obviously you are supposed to keep really still....You do not want the needle to go anywhere near the fetus, and I just literally jumped, because it was really shocking....It hurt a bit, it wasn't hugely painful. It was the fact that it was this kind of, a major sort of pop through, you know. Pressure, pressure, pressure, pressure, pop" (55).

Overall, 97 percent of people who have amniocentesis either report no pain or describe the pain as "bearable," similar to having a blood sample taken (56). Talking beforehand with the doctor performing your amniocentesis is helpful, because it is important that you have a lot of faith and trust in their skill level. If possible, have the procedure done at a large centre, where they perform a lot of prenatal testing and get a lot of practice. Lastly, take advantage of other anxiety-reducing techniques, like mindfulness or prayer, focused breathing, or just closing your eyes.

Steph used positive affirmations to help manage her anxiety. She describes her method of placing "positive affirmations under my keyboard where only I can see them. I have one that I actually wrote when I was pregnant with Grace. I was about six or eight weeks pregnant with her and I started bleeding. While I was waiting to talk to my doctor I was at my desk and no one was in the office so I wrote on a little Post-It note: "Stay with me, little one." I just kept it and I still have it under plastic at my desk. I also have an image made by another baby loss mom that says, "I will carry my baby to term and I will bring my baby home from the hospital healthy and happy." I say it on my way to work. I say it all the time. I keep one in my wallet for when I open my wallet. I keep one in the car. I keep it at my desk at work. I just have them everywhere."

Charlotte also talks about the struggle to keep her anxiety in check. In her words: "For me, that's the most difficult thing about pregnancy after a loss. You know that your stress is not helping the baby, but of course it is the most natural thing in the world to be stressed. And there's no line, there's absolutely no line that you can draw and say, okay, this is safe worry, this is not safe worry, because it does not exist. Every day you have to negotiate what is reasonable for you. And some of it is sticking your head in the sand and saying of course, everything's going to be fine. And some of it is being overcautious and going with that."

Week 16

Week 16 sees your baby measure somewhere between four and five inches (10 and 13 centimetres) long. Your baby is still growing steadily and gaining weight and is starting to look more and more like someone you would recognize. It is still too early for distinctive facial features, all babies kinda look the same at this stage, but those little changes that make you you are starting to happen!

Because you are beginning to show, now is a good time to start documenting yourself during pregnancy if you have not done so already. There are lots of ways to do this, from keeping a journal to taking weekly pictures of your growing baby bump. I did not do it during my subsequent pregnancies, I just did not feel comfortable. I was still at the stage where I hated pictures of myself, especially of my pregnant self. Those pictures represented the naive, happy person I once was. The person before I lost my sons. Author Francesca Cox, who created the Still Standing magazine blog, has another idea. She suggests these shameless selfies are a great way to bond with your baby and feel better about yourself.

10 Reasons to Document Your Pregnancy After Loss with **Shameless Selfies**

August 23, 2014, by Francesca Cox, reprinted with permission from http://www.pregnancyafterlosssupport.com/10-reasons-document-pregnancy-loss-shameless-selfies/

I am not a big fan of selfies, unless of course it has to do with the miracle of carrying new life into this world and celebrating it with shameless shots of your ever growing bump! You might feel totally out of your comfort zone, and that is to be expected. Few women feel glamorous when pregnant (does anyone besides Gisele?), but the truth is, a woman is almost never more radiant than when she is carrying new life. Regardless, the benefits below of documenting this time in your life have little to do with glamour and have everything to do with healing, self-care and bonding.

1 Documenting this time in your life can be therapeutic and healing on so many levels. In retrospect you will be able to say, "I celebrated my pregnancy, as hard as it was…" (of course there are SO many ways to celebrate your pregnancy! This is just one.)

2 It gives you a chance to have something to celebrate NOW. The thing I hear the most from Pregnancy After Loss mamas (and something I often thought myself) is that they will be able to breathe/be happy/celebrate once the baby is alive, and in their arms. I get it, I really do. I felt the exact same way, but give yourself the liberty to celebrate something before that milestone—that so often feels eons away.

3 Watch your growing belly. It gives you the chance see how it grows so quickly from month to month.

4 Gain your confidence back. After experiencing a loss, confidence is often the first thing to go. Personally, I felt like my body had betrayed me and my first child. Unless you live with chronic pain and illness, or grow up close to someone who deals with chronic pain and illness, you instinctively trust your body to do what it's supposed to do, especially during pregnancy. Documenting your pregnancy with pictures can help you restore some of that lost confidence and give you some visible markers of what your body can do, and has done.

5 Something to look forward to. I started to really enjoy documenting my pregnancy with E, our last baby. I hardly had any preggo pictures with my first "rainbow." That particularly made me sad, but it was very reflective of how I felt of the entire nine or so months—petrified of something going wrong, anxious, and leery of celebrating or being too happy about it or even crazier—jinxing it. I decided to make this last pregnancy one I would shamelessly celebrate.

6 Bonding with baby time. If it's one thing that pregnancy after loss moms feel, it is probably guilt. Guilty about being pregnant again "too soon," guilty about buying something for baby, guilty about being happy, or relieved, or whatever. Guilt, guilt, guilt. The relentless guilt often leads mama to distance herself from the baby, in a survival kind of way, but also in an I'm-not-over-my-loss-and-do-not-know-how-to-embrace-this-new-pregnancy kind of way too. Snapping shots of the two of you will give you some bonding time, if you are struggling with bonding with this new baby, which by the way, is totally and completely normal.

7 Your bump is freakin' beautiful. Has anyone told you yet? Because it is. It is an absolute wonder, actually. Think about it. You are growing fingers, toes, a beating heart, tiny lungs, a human brain that will think thoughts and learn to speak one or two languages. Please, dear mama, do not underestimate your beauty, your courage, and all the magic that pregnancy (especially after loss!) entails.

8 Get gussied up! Okay, so realistically you might not be in the mood for dress-up and heels, but taking selfies once a month or once a week can give you an excuse to try on a new lipstick, shop for a new maternity shirt or try a five minute hair style you spotted on Pinterest one afternoon.

9 If you plan on sharing your pictures on Instagram or a social media, without probably realizing it, you are creating your community. You are drawing people in, and sharing this time in your life will give you the support you need the most to celebrate this beautiful and intensely bittersweet time in your life.

10 You document things going on in your life, while you are pregnant, that you might otherwise not remember vividly. Because I chose to take a picture, I remember that I was exactly 16 weeks on the day my brother-in-law and sister-in-law tied the knot, a wedding that both me and my husband got to be a part of. It was a pretty special day for everyone. While shopping for a dress that was maternity friendly was not the highlight of my pregnancy, sharing that time with close family, and this sweet girl on the way was. So, so special.

Week 17: Get Crafty!

Here is a great way to burn off a little nervous energy. While there are lots of kick counters on the market, making your own can be a great way to help bond with this baby, and you can personalize it however you choose. I found my kick-counter bracelet especially helpful during those early months when I wasn't feeling the baby move often enough to do formal kick counting, but still needed that reassurance. Also, unlike an app, my kick-counter bracelet was a way to reassure my husband that everything was okay. It allowed him to see what was going on and know that I had felt the baby move recently.

Here's what you need:

» Memory wire or durable elastic string

» Numbered beads from one to 12

» A charm that has meaning to you

» A lobster clasp—make sure the lobster clasp is large enough the beads will not pass through the centre of the clasp

» 36 beads of approximately the same size as your numbered beads

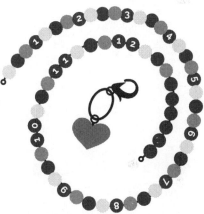

Here's what to do:

String the beads in sequence along the memory wire, so you have three standard beads, then a number, sequenced from one to 12. Each plain bead marks a 15-minute interval. This will make your bracelet. Depending on the size of your beads, you may need to wrap the bracelet around your wrist more than once. Attach the lobster clasp to the charm so that it creates a movable place-marker you can attach to the bracelet.

Here is how it works:

Imagine you are at work one morning and you feel baby move. You check the time, and it's 10:15 am. Just move your charm to the spot on the bracelet that indicates 10:15, which is one bead past the #10 bead. Later, after lunch, you feel another kick.

The time is 12:40, so you move the charm to three beads past the 12 (the closest time on the bracelet). Now, whenever you feel anxious, a quick glance at your wrist reminds you of when you last felt a kick.

Because the beads often make these bracelets quite a bit larger than your wrist (I had to wrap mine around twice), they also make great necklaces for your son or daughter when they are old enough. The bracelets also make nice gifts for friends who are pregnant.

At this stage of the pregnancy, your baby's eyes are continuing to form, but they have moved more or less to the part of the face where they belong. Babies can also react to sounds, although they are not able to hear anything distinguishable, just loud noises. If you pop a balloon near your belly, they might jump, but it is still too early for playing Mozart!

This is roughly the earliest you might begin to feel your baby move. While it is normal to feel movement earlier in second and later pregnancies, not feeling the baby move just yet is completely normal too. Whenever you reach this exciting milestone, for loss moms it can be especially bittersweet. Your mind will be filled with memories of your last pregnancy and guilt that if you had only been more careful in this important task, your circumstances might have been different. Maybe you told your doctor about decreased movement and she did not seem to listen. Or maybe you lost track yourself. When you first feel your baby move is a good time to work on banishing those thoughts so they do not make your anxiety worse. Most doctors tell you to start kick counting later in the pregnancy (sometime between weeks 24 and 29). However, even if kicks are not regular at this stage, every time you feel them can be a reassurance that your baby is still okay.

Certainly Steph found this to be true. When she was 22 weeks along, she talked about how she was "starting to feel the kicks and rolls, so now when I do not feel them, I start to get nervous. And I'll sit there, especially if I'm at work, and I'll think, have I felt the baby move yet? I do not remember! And I'll sit there and I'll think really hard, you know, think, think, think. And then I'll feel a kick and I'll go back about my day." However, at this stage, the kicks still are not regular and can be hard to track. When Steph was feeling anxious over not feeling her baby move, she went to the doctor because, while she could hear the heartbeat on the home Doppler, she couldn't feel movement. As she says, they went in "and found her on the Doppler and on the sonogram. It turns out my placenta is in the front, so when she kicks to the front I do not feel it." You can read more about kick counting in chapter eight.

Week 18

Around this week, your baby truly becomes an individual. Of course your baby has always been unique, but this week is about the time that fingerprints develop. Everyone has their own unique fingerprint, and even identical twins do not share fingerprints.

7

WEEKS 19-24

Week 19

At yet another week closer, you may be feeling especially anxious as you approach the 20-week scan. Plenty of first-time moms see the 20-week scan as the time they will confirm the baby's sex. They plan the baby's sex reveal party. They get the cool 3D ultrasound photos. Loss moms see it differently. This may be a week of painful reminders of your last pregnancy. You might worry that the baby will have the same medical condition as your last. You might fear going into the same hospital unit where you found out your baby had died. In many cases of pregnancy loss, it was an ultrasound that confirmed your baby's death. For this reason, ultrasound has a very different meaning for you than it would for another mother.

However, ultrasounds are also used to confirm that your baby is healthy and growing normally. Because of this, many parents report feeling very conflicted. On one hand, they need that ultrasound to know their baby is okay. On the other hand, they are afraid to look (52). Regina talked about this the night before her anatomical ultrasound: "They'll be checking the baby and also, checking my placenta and stuff like that. I am afraid I'll regress tomorrow, that there will be a cord or placenta issue or things that I did not even know about before. I just hope these people know exactly what they are doing and what happened the first time. Sometimes they are so busy, busy, busy. It's a big hospital and they are very specialized, but at the same time I just hope that they pay attention to what they are doing."

Due to this conflict, you might want to prepare yourself for flashbacks, especially if your ultrasound will take place at the same location. A flashback is a particular sensation that the traumatic experience is happening all over again. Flashbacks come without warning and can be triggered by seemingly harmless things. If you can, ensure that the sonographer is aware of your past history (your doctor or midwife can help with this). You can also take a few moments before the ultrasound to remind yourself that this is a different time, and a different pregnancy. This is called debriefing. Try doing something to consciously make yourself aware of the different circumstances, like taking a different route to the hospital or wearing a new outfit that you did not own during your last pregnancy. These small actions can help to differentiate your past experiences from this one. Just knowing that ultrasounds are a common time for flashbacks and emotions to come to the surface helps, so you will not be alarmed if you experience them. They are common in pregnancies after a loss. Do not be surprised if your anxiety does not diminish after the ultrasound, either. In one study of high-risk pregnancies, the only group of high-risk moms who saw an increase in anxiety despite a reassuring ultrasound were loss moms (52).

What can you expect at a 20-week ultrasound? The mid-trimester ultrasound is also sometimes called a Level 2 scan because it is more detailed than the Level 1 scan done around week 12. If you were not able to accurately tell the sex of your baby at the 12-week scan, they can often tell by the 20-week scan.

Whether or not you want to find out the sex of your child is up to you. For me, in my first pregnancy after a loss, I wanted to know. With my second pregnancy, I did not. In the case of my daughter, I was very concerned that I would be disappointed that she was a girl. And truth be told, I was. Being disappointed that you are having a girl when you lost a boy is normal, and vice versa. Being pregnant with a boy after you have lost a girl can result in disappointment too. For me, knowing the sex gave me several more weeks to get used to the idea that I was having a girl. It helped me to choose her name, which made bonding with her easier. Instead of "the baby" or more often "this baby," she was now Rebecca. She was Nate and Sam's little sister.

However, when I became pregnant with my son, I did not want to know whether he was a boy or a girl. I was more comfortable with not knowing. Bonding with him was less of an issue because I had already had a successful pregnancy. Of course, you do not need to decide now. In most instances, you will have several more ultrasounds between now and when you deliver, so there will be other opportunities to find out. Depending on your medical condition, your pregnancy, and your anxiety levels, you may even have an ultrasound every week for the rest of the pregnancy. If you want to have ultrasound scans to ease your mind, talk you your doctor about how often this can be done. Also ask how often they think you might need a scan based on your medical history. There may be other ways to reassure you that the pregnancy is going well without having to have a full ultrasound.

Week 20

You have now officially reached the midpoint of pregnancy. As you probably already know, this is an arbitrary number because babies do not magically come on their due dates. As someone who has had a loss, it is quite likely you will deliver a little early. All the same, use the midpoint as an excuse for a mini-celebration.

At week 20, several interesting things start happening to your baby. The tiniest bones in the human body, the ones in the inner ear, form and harden around this week (44). If you are prone to having hairy babies, the first hair on the scalp starts to become visible (14). Also beginning to form is the vernix caseosa. Believe it or not, that's from the Latin for "cheese-like varnish" (caseosa, same root word as the protein casein). It is made up of the skin your baby will start to slough off, lanugo (the soft body hair newborns often have), and other skin secretions (57). Doctors are not completely clear on the purpose of vernix caseosa other than to protect your baby from their watery uterine environment and possibly from meconium and infection. Only humans are known to have this substance—no other mammals have it. Any vernix caseosa remaining on your baby when she is born will be wiped off or cleaned at her first bath.

If you are tracking movements or kick counts already, your baby will be active only about 10 to 30 percent of the time, but will have movements of about once a minute during these active periods (14). Most of these will be far too small to feel. So if you are not feeling much movement yet, that is completely normal. There may be a lot more going on that you are just not detecting.

Names

Now that you are midway through your pregnancy, you might be starting to think about names. Naming a child, and especially a second or third child, is increasingly difficult. Years ago, people used a small set of names and recycled them often, so there were entire classrooms of little Marys and Johns. Now, choosing a name seems like an emotionally fraught decision. But giving your child a name (or names, one for a boy, one for a girl, if you have decided to keep the sex secret), can help you feel connected to this baby. When you are choosing a name for a child after a loss, you can run into some challenges, especially if you want to honour your lost child.

One of the few things I remember about being in labour with my sons was a discussion I had with my husband over their names. We had planned to name them Nathaniel Thomas and Samuel James, but were unsure what to do. I asked him if we should go ahead with naming them, even though they were stillborn, or whether we should "save" the names for our future children. The nurse piped up and said, "I think you should name them. Those are *their* names!" I am so glad she said that, and I am glad I gave them their names.

For a variety of reasons, including culture, you may want to give your child the same or a similar name as the baby you lost. In some cultures, naming a child after a deceased family member is common, and even expected. In others, naming a child after a deceased family member is considered bad luck. Whichever you choose, you can expect strong feedback from people who are completely against the idea. One mother wrote to The Name Lady asking for her advice on naming a child after her husband. She had done that for her first son, who died at birth, and was wondering if she could do the same for her second son. Would her second son also be a Junior, and was having two sons with the same legal name going to cause problems, even if her first son had died. The Name Lady answered with advice and some wise words:

My sympathies to you and your husband. A name that's associated with the loss of a child can be a painful reminder of hopes and futures unfulfilled. When the departed child is a namesake there can be an added sting, as the name symbolizes the family traditions that the child won't be able to carry on. It sounds like you and your husband are very attached to the idea of having a Junior. It must seem cruel to have to give up that dream. Is giving a new baby the exact same name as a brother who died legal? Yes. Is it common? No—at least, not in modern America.

Once upon a time, though, childhood mortality rates were terribly high. Prior to the mid-19th century, the average American family lost at least one child. In colonial times, many families followed a tradition of naming their next baby after a child who had passed away. For example, Paul Revere had two brothers named Thomas and two sisters named Elizabeth. The names were chosen as homage and remembrance for the lost siblings. In your case, if you choose, your new son's name could act as a double namesake, honoring both his father and his late brother.

> *As for whether your son should be called Junior, that's a gray area. Some will tell you that the suffix III is technically correct, in that he would be the third in your family to bear this name. Others believe that suffixes "move up" when one in the order of succession passes on, making Jr. the proper designation.*
>
> *So how should you choose? I say follow your heart. If you feel that a III suffix would honor the memory of the baby you lost, use that. But if you feel that naming your son III would be a painful reminder of the baby you lost and raise awkward questions from people you and your son meet in the future, you should feel perfectly comfortable giving your son the exact same name as his deceased brother, Junior included.*
>
> *The whole point of family names and homages is to promote good feelings within the family: closeness, continuity, love, solace. Choose the designation that feels the best to you* (58).

Certainly, giving your child the exact same name can come with legal hiccups, especially if your child received a birth certificate. And there will be some people who give you strong negative feedback. However, if this name is important to you and your family, then why not? After all, George Foreman named all five of his sons George Foreman (Jr., III, IV, V, and IV), and they are all alive!

However, there are other ways to honour your child. You could give them a similar name, one that is less likely to attract criticism. You could use an international variation on a given name, such as using the Italian Giovanni or the Scottish Ian to honour a child named John. Instead of Jacob, consider the Spanish Diego or the French Jacques. You could also give your child a middle name that is the same. Another common option is to give the child the same initials, so to honour Nathaniel Thomas we could have named our daughter Nicola Theresa. Or for a truly hidden meaning, use a baby name book to find names with the same meaning. For example, Tabitha means gazelle. Other names that also mean gazelle are Ayelet, Leah, and Rasha. Because this is a little more obscure than the other options, you can keep this as a secret tribute and only reveal it to those who will be sympathetic.

As I mentioned earlier, we have a lot more choice in baby names now and there is more value placed on having a "unique" name. We are no longer limited to just naming our children Mary or John, but can choose a name that reflects the many cultures and traditions we are a part of. Steph had an unusual perspective on how names for our deceased children have changed over time. Not only did she experience a loss, but so did her mother. Before Steph was born, her mother had two sons who were stillborn. She went on to have Steph and Steph's (living) brother. Steph noticed that one difference between her mother's generation and her own is the role her own son plays in the family compared to that of her dead brothers'. All three of her brothers were named after her father, which made it harder to distinguish her living brother from the two who died. As she says, "They were not as open about it [her mother's losses]. Two of them were born and all had my dad's name. My oldest brother has my dad's name too. They did not have their own names. They did not have all the things we have for our babies."

Week 21

By week 21, your baby has started to eat her amniotic fluid. Yuck! This is not really for nutritional purposes. Your placenta provides the nourishment your baby needs. Instead, you can consider this swallowing of amniotic fluid as practice to get the intestines ready to ingest breast milk or formula after she is born. What does amniotic fluid taste like? I really do not want to find out, but some researchers suggest it tastes a lot like whatever you have been eating. If you have a craving for eggs, your baby will like eggs. If it is your mom's spinach lasagna, that will be something your baby loves too. How did they test this? They gave the moms carrot juice to drink, either while they were pregnant or while they were breastfeeding. Later, when the babies had cereal, they blended the cereal with carrot juice to see how they liked it. The babies whose mothers drank carrot juice, either while pregnant or while breastfeeding, liked the carrot-juice-blended cereal better than the mothers who did not drink carrot juice (59). You can use this as an excuse to try a new food this week!

Week 22

At week 22, your baby weighs about one pound (or 500 grams). Most women also are able to feel movement by this point, although no need to panic if you still cannot feel a thing. Depending on where the placenta is located, it just may be harder for you to feel movements. Starting around now, you may also be able to feel those little kicks from the outside. This can be a great way to get your partner, friends, and family involved. Some people also have trouble at this time with others, including coworkers, friends, or even complete strangers, wanting to touch their belly. I never had this issue, but if it makes you uncomfortable, speak up! It is perfectly okay to tell someone, "Sorry but this is something I want to keep to myself."

Week 23

By week 23, your baby is continuing to grow and put on weight. For much of the rest of the pregnancy, the changes will be small and will reflect this increased growth period both in height/length and weight. This is also around the time practitioners will recommend you consider childbirth classes. There are many different types of classes, and choosing to take one is entirely up to you. Some women who are pregnant after a loss would rather not. They have experienced labour before, and taking a childbirth class will inevitably involve awkward moments with pregnant moms who do not want to hear your story.

However, there can be benefits too. If you hope or expect to have a radically different delivery from your last birth, classes can help you prepare. For example, if you are hoping for a vaginal birth when your last was a cesarean (or the other way around), or if you know that due to complications you will likely have a cesarean, you can learn more about what is involved. You may also have had a very early birth last time and didn't have the chance to take prenatal classes. You might be giving birth at a different hospital, or your hospital has renovated since your last birth and new birthing equipment (such as birthing beds or pools) are available.

If you are concerned about how you will answer questions from other new moms in the class, it can be helpful to have a conversation with the instructor beforehand. Call and ask to speak to him or her, let them know your circumstances, and ask how they want it handled. They may offer to let the class know in advance so that you do not have to explain yourself. You can also practice how you want to answer, whether that is to not tell people at all or to simply state things as matter-of-factly as you can. One solution for avoiding these situations is to take an online class, which some hospitals now offer. If this seems right for you, it can be a good option.

Charlotte talked about how she met a lot of mothers through her first prenatal class, but that with this pregnancy, she does not feel comfortable. "I do not feel like I belong in those circles because in many ways I am the same as other first-time mothers, but in other ways I'm not. I feel like I am [the] walking wounded. If I were to go into those groups to do those classes again and talk about my story, it would just freak them all out. These mothers are freaked out enough as it is, and I would go in and say, 'oh, by the way, the night before your baby's about to come out, they could just die, and there won't be any reason for it and you won't see it coming. But I am pretty sure it won't happen to you. Although, you know, that's what I thought, ha ha.' I am hoping that after the baby's born, I can maybe fit in with the new moms that way. Because they'll have their babies by then, they'll be secure, my story won't be such a threat. But it's pretty isolating at the moment."

It can be useful to have a tour of the labour and delivery suites before you go in, and this is often done as part of a prenatal class. You can also ask your doctor to arrange a private tour because, as you can imagine, going back to the same location will bring back powerful memories. I was lucky enough to have the charge nurse offer to take me through the labour and delivery suites, and while I wasn't ready to see the room where I actually gave birth to my twins, seeing one of the rooms helped me feel prepared to go in there and not panic. Physical location can be a strong trigger and one that crops up unexpectedly. I remember going in for something and the nurses asked for a urine sample. There was one toilet in the assessment area and I had used that same toilet when the boys died. I did not feel like I could ask the nurses to use another toilet.

Even though Regina was unlikely to deliver at the same hospital where she lost Jacob, she described the need to go back. "I do not know why I feel the need to go and visit the room where I delivered Jacob. I haven't been there since it happened. It is just something I need to do. I can't explain why. It is like I need to go. I asked if I could go and I can as long as it is empty. I mentioned it to Scott and he said we'll see. I do not know, I need to see it and spend a few minutes there."

Maeve describes the first time she went back to the same assessment unit: "Over a year and I had actually forgotten where it was. I really had blocked it out. But as soon as we went through the doors I remembered it very clearly. We went to the waiting room and on one side there were already people sitting. On the other side was where I sat with Gavin when we were waiting to find out about Cord. So I couldn't sit there again. But I was really busting for the toilet. I couldn't go with only one bathroom. I couldn't go into the bathroom because that was where we found out that Cord had passed. When they couldn't find him on the ultrasound in the maternity assessment ward, they couldn't find him on the Doppler, and they did not tell me, but I knew he had died. I knew it. They said they would take me over to radiography where they do the formal scan, but I thought to myself, they already know he is dead but they are getting me away from this room. But I went to that toilet in that bedroom before we went off to that room. So last Friday when we were there, even though I was busting, I couldn't go back to that toilet. I couldn't sit in that same chair in the waiting room."

Viability

Viability is a tricky concept and one that is constantly changing. Around this time, it will be determined that your baby is viable, and that has different meanings depending on the jurisdiction you live in. The definition also changes over time and can vary from hospital to hospital. Legal definitions also differ from medical ones. This can be frustrating to laypeople who want medicine to have clear-cut answers. It can be hurtful to women who watch as their baby born at 23 weeks is not saved, but hear of another born in a different hospital who was.

It can be challenging for researchers, too, because the different definitions make it hard to compare statistics. If a baby is deemed viable at 20 weeks in one state but only at 25 weeks in another, how do you measure which hospital is more successful in treating babies? In the United States the legal definition of a viable baby varies from state to state, but is usually between 20 and 24 weeks. One common definition of fetal viability is this: "The ability of a fetus to survive outside of the womb. Historically, a fetus was considered to be capable of living at the end of gestational week 20 when the mother had felt fetal movement (quickening) and the fetal heart tones could be auscultated with a fetoscope. In actuality, even with prompt and intensive neonatal support, a preterm fetus of less than 23 weeks' gestation has little chance of surviving outside of the womb" (57). If you had a mid-trimester loss or a very preterm infant, however, passing the point of viability can be a reason to celebrate. If the baby had been born before this period, there would be little that could be done. From this point on, with each passing week, your baby's chances of surviving outside the womb improve. That is worth celebrating!

Certainly a lot of women who have had a loss are very aware of the milestone of viability. Maeve lives in Australia, where babies are considered viable at 24 weeks. She talks about managing her anxiety when she did not feel a lot of movements, but was before the period where her baby was considered viable. She says, "I am more hyperaware now. I've certainly had periods of up to 48 hours where I was convinced the baby was dead, and the only reason I did not go to hospital was because I knew I was before 24 weeks and so if I was really in fetal distress there was nothing they could really do. Gavin would say to me, 'Well if you are that scared, why don't you go to hospital?' And I'd say 'no, it's just emotional.' But I'd still be thinking to myself, if I go there, what am I going to do? I am just going to have to give birth to this baby that's going to die anyway."

Week 24

Your baby is still growing and gaining about five or six ounces (150 grams) a week at this stage. It does not sound like much, but unless there is a concern about having an overly large baby—if you are diabetic, for example—then each one of those ounces is helpful for the baby's survival. Around week 24 is also when your doctor or midwife will do a gestational diabetes test, sometimes called a glucose screening test. This is a two-stage test, although you only have to do the second stage if your first one indicates there might be an issue.

In the first test, you will be asked to drink an ultra-sweet orange liquid exactly one hour before your blood is taken. The blood will be sent to the lab to determine your blood sugar level, and if it is high, you will be asked to take a second test (60). Some people find the sugary drink a little too sweet for their taste, so my doctor suggested drinking it cold. I have no idea if that made it any more palatable.

If you are asked to do the second test, called the glucose tolerance test, it will be fairly similar to the first, but with a few important differences. You will be asked to fast for three hours (not eat or drink anything) before taking the super-sweet drink, and the drink will be of a higher glucose concentration. Often, you will take the drink first thing in the morning, before you have had breakfast. Again, you will have to wait exactly one hour before having your blood taken. In both tests the timing is very important, so you might want to show up an hour early at the lab where your blood will be drawn and drink it there, then enjoy your one hour in the waiting room with a good book. Also, if the lab is busy and you notice you are getting close to your time, speak up and let someone know.

Maeve was diagnosed with gestational diabetes in her pregnancy after a loss. She did not have it during her first pregnancy. She describes how she felt guilty about her diagnosis because she felt she was doing something wrong:

"At first, I felt really bad about it, actually. It's apparently a common reaction, I guess. I felt really worried about what to eat. It is a lot of work. I am hungry. We are really busy and I am finding myself having to prepare a lot of easy snacking foods. I have to check my blood four times a day and I have to not eat for two hours after a meal, which is really hard for me. I have been going to the hospital a lot as it is, and now I have extra appointments with the gestational diabetes." After her diagnosis she had two appointments, one for a group diabetes education session and another with the dietician at the hospital. The group education session was held in the same room as the prenatal education classes she had taken with her son, Cord, so that added another element of stress. She added, *"I went in there thinking, I do not want to talk about Cord. I do not want to bring that up here. I was really highly uncomfortable and stressed going in once I realized it was the same environment. We were all worried about pricking our fingers for the first time and she told us how to do it. Then she said, 'If you do not do it properly and you do not get any blood that means you won't be able to take home your babies.' I just went off! I just felt really stressed in there and really unhappy."*

Maeve found it frustrating when she wasn't able to get her blood glucose levels into the normal range. She felt she was already doing everything right, like exercising and eating properly. It was simply another added stress on top of an already stressful pregnancy. In the end, Maeve felt more at peace with her diagnosis and was able to feel calmer about managing her blood sugar levels. As she says, "These last couple days have been happy because all of my fasting ones have been less than 5.5, which is where they are meant to be. All of my post-meal ones have been less than 7, which is what they are meant to be." Even at the diabetes education class, in the end she felt pretty good, "even though I was very uncomfortable there, just to be amongst all those other pregnant women and not mention Cord and just act like them. Not like I hid him or anything. They asked everyone if this was their first pregnancy. For nobody it was. Everybody was at least number two, including me, and that is as far as it got with that question. That is a big step for me."

If you are diagnosed with gestational diabetes, you are not alone. Approximately seven percent of women get this common condition during pregnancy, and while it may mean some lifestyle changes, most women do not go on to develop Type 2

Diabetes (sometimes called non-insulin dependent). However, you will be at risk for this condition, so you will have to be tested again after your pregnancy is over. In most cases you will not have to take any medication to control your blood sugar, as diet and exercise changes will be enough. Your doctor or midwife should refer you to a diabetes educator or a dietician for advice on how to make these changes. There are some great resources available for gestational diabetes on the **MedlinePlus** website at **http://www.nlm.nih.gov/medlineplus/diabetesandpregnancy.html**.

8

WEEKS 25-29

Week 25

At around week 25, when their nostrils open, your baby will start to take practice breaths. Your practitioner will likely be watching for these practice breaths on ultrasounds if you are having these regularly. It will still be a while before your baby is able to breathe on their own, but these practice breaths can help the doctor to determine how ready the lungs are for birth. Another exciting development around this time is that your baby's heartbeat can be heard with a regular stethoscope and not just on the Doppler. If you have a stethoscope, or have access to one, give it a try!

Week 26

At this stage in your pregnancy, your baby weighs around 32 ounces (900 grams) (44). You may also begin to feel the baby hiccupping! This week at your doctor's appointment, ask about whether you are current or need to be given a booster of the Tdap (short for tetanus, diphtheria, and pertussis) immunization. I mentioned the importance of protecting yourself and your baby from infectious diseases earlier, but this particular vaccine is best given between weeks 27 and 36 of pregnancy, so it is worth it to remind you here. You will also want to make sure your spouse, family members, and anyone who'll be in contact with you or your baby have had their recommended vaccinations. The Center for Disease Control and the American College of Obstetricians and Gynecologists recommend Tdap booster for good reason: Whooping cough is one of the most easily preventable bacterial infections and can cause serious harm to pregnant women and their babies (61).

I do not write this based only on the medical evidence, which is overwhelmingly in favour of immunization. I write this based also on personal experience. One of the scariest things that can happen in a pregnancy after a loss happened to me. I still do not know for certain if it was whooping cough or influenza that got me, but I started to cough. A lot.

At first, I thought it was a simple run-of-the-mill cold. I mentioned it to my obstetrician, and he thought it was simply that my tired body was taking longer than usual to get over a cold. I also mentioned it to my family doctor, and he told me the same thing. Then, one Tuesday after work, I felt a little feverish. I put my daughter to bed at her usual time, took my temperature and some Tylenol and went to bed early. I knew I was coming down with something. By the middle of the night, my fever had jumped and I was having difficulty breathing. I woke up in a panic and realized I had to get to the hospital fast. This was more than a simple cold. My husband had to stay with our daughter while she slept, and I took a cab to the hospital. I was coughing up blood and my fever continued to rise. Fortunately, my obstetrician happened to be the one on call. I sat in the triage area as they brought up a portable x-ray machine to look at my chest. My bacterial infection had become pneumonia. I was sent home with a prescription for antibiotics and plenty of fluids and rest.

If this were the end of the story, it would be a good tale, and nothing more. But it is not. The antibiotics I was given were not controlling the infection. My fever continued to rise. By noon the next day, I was back in hospital. They checked my oxygen levels and they were below 90 (normal is between 90 and 95, slightly higher when you are pregnant). To a mother who lost her first children to hypoxia, or a lack of oxygen, nothing could be more frightening. I was now being given oxygen through a cannula (the little tube that goes against your nose) and antibiotics through an IV. Despite this, my oxygen levels continued to drop. Due to the lack of oxygen and high fever, I was delirious and not able to think straight. Fortunately, a smart nurse made a good decision. She called downstairs to the intensive care unit, where I was evaluated by a respiratory therapist and an intensivist, a specialist in critical care medicine. I was moved from the obstetrical ward to the intensive care unit where I spent five days hooked up to a continuous positive airway pressure (CPAP) machine that would help me breathe. I was given more antibiotics, and a special catheter was put in to deliver emergency medications to my heart, in case I needed resuscitating. Too sick to be fully aware of what was going on, doctors discussed with my husband what to do in case my son started to show signs of fetal distress. They reassured him that at 28 weeks pregnant, they could perform an emergency cesarean section on me if necessary, but that they would monitor me closely. It was a very frightening time. I was given morphine for the pain, which was constant, and eventually they had to put in a chest tube—the back is punctured to allow accumulated fluid in the lungs to drain out. But after draining over 50 ounces (1.5 litres) of fluid from my lungs, the pain had grown too much for me and they had to take it out. Eventually, I was moved out of intensive care and back to the obstetrical unit, where I continued to recover for another five days.

Because of this experience, and because of my job, I am passionate about making sure everyone is protected from illness by becoming immunized. I can appreciate that a lot of people are scared of needles, or think that illness will not happen to them, or simply forget to keep their immunizations up to date. I can also appreciate that, having trusted the medical establishment with your last pregnancy, it can be hard to do so again. If you have any questions about vaccinations, please talk to your doctor or a public health nurse. They have great decision aids that can help you weigh the pros and cons associated with getting your vaccine. This is one of those topics about which there is far too much unreliable and dangerous information circulating on the Internet. It is so important to get immunization information from a trusted source.

For more information on the safety of the flu vaccine during pregnancy, see the **Center for Disease Control**'s website at **http://www.cdc.gov/flu/protect/vaccine/qa_vacpregnant.html**. For more information on the safety of the Tdap vaccine during pregnancy, see the **Organization of Teratology Information Specialists**' fact sheet at **http://www.mothertobaby.org/files/Tdap.pdf**. Another great source for reliable information on vaccinations is **MedlinePlus.gov**.

*Just to be clear about which vaccinations I received, I did get the flu shot that year as I do every year. The flu shot does not provide 100 percent protection, so it is still possible that I got the flu despite protecting myself with a vaccine. I did not have a Tdap booster, because at that time boosters were not done for adults, you simply received the vaccines on schedule as a child. Because whooping cough is making a resurgence, adults whose vaccine protection had waned are no longer protected by herd immunity.

Is it CRAAP?

In my day job, I teach nursing students how to evaluate information, including information found online. I like a method called the CRAAP test, mostly because it makes for a catchy acronym, but also because it is a simple way to decide whether information found on the Internet is worth taking seriously (62).

CRAAP stands for **Currency, Relevance, Accuracy, Authority** and **Purpose**. Keeping these five things in mind as you read through any information, but especially information online, can help you to look at what you're seeing with a critical eye.

Currency [1]

Material found online can quickly become out of date. Websites fall out of use, are no longer maintained, or disappear altogether. The following criteria will help you judge the currency of a website:

» Is there a date of publication or last update? When was the page created?
» Do the links work?
» Is the page maintained on a regular basis?

Relevance

You are unique, and so are your needs. Sometimes information is written with another audience in mind.

» Does the information relate to you or answer your question?
» Who is the intended audience and is the information at an appropriate level (not too basic or advanced) for your needs?
» Does the site claim to be comprehensive and how does it meet those claims?

Accuracy

There are no regulations, standards, or systems in place to ensure that information on the web is correct. Judging the accuracy of information is important when utilizing Internet resources.

» Is the information correct? Can it be verified from other sources?
» Is the information cited, and cited by reputable peer-reviewed journals?
» Are there spelling, grammatical, or typographical errors?
» Has the information been refereed?

Authority

Anyone has the ability to publish information on the Internet. This does not mean they are qualified experts. The following questions will help you decide if the website is an authoritative source:

» Who is the author of the page? What are their credentials?

» What institution are they affiliated with? Is it a reputable institution?

» Is there an email address or other contact information?

» What does the domain name tell you about the source? Watch for similarly named sites that have slightly different domain names.

Purpose

It should be clear why the information on the website is being made available. Knowing and understanding the purpose of information is key to conducting high-quality research.

» Is this information meant to teach? Inform? Persuade? Entertain?

» Do the authors/sponsors make their intentions or purpose clear?

» Is the information fact? Opinion? Propaganda?

» What other websites are linked to this one?

» Is there advertising on the site? What is being advertised?

» Does the point of view appear objective and impartial?

» Are there political, ideological, cultural, religious, institutional, or personal biases?

[1] *This has been adapted, largely verbatim, from Queen's Library's own page on Evaluating Web Sources at: http://library.queensu.ca/inforef/tutorials/qcat/evalint. htm. Accessed October 26, 2016.*

Week 27

A couple of important changes happen to your baby over the next few weeks. First of all, your baby's hearing will start to develop to the point where he can recognize voices from outside the womb. As a means of helping bond with your child (and with you!), now is a good time to have your partner read to you—and to your baby. This can be a challenge if it brings up painful reminders of your last pregnancy. Depending on how he is feeling about it, you can read the same books as you did during your last pregnancy, or you can get new ones. If you are still not at the stage where you are comfortable buying things for your baby, you can borrow books from the library or a friend. If your partner is not ready for this step, you could also ask other important people in your life to try reading to your baby. Reading aloud is something we do not do very often as adults, but it has a lot of benefit for us and our children. Try reading in front of a mirror, or making silly voices. Most of all, try to have fun with it. Reading to your baby in utero may not give them a leg up in school, but it does have lots of other benefits. Through reading, you will be practising your own speaking voice, developing a sense of yourself as a parent, and sharing your baby with your partner and other family members.

Week 28

Signs of Preterm Labour to Watch For: (18)

» Regular contractions of the uterus. These are different from Braxton-Hicks contractions because they are regular and often more painful than Braxton-Hicks contractions.

» A low dull backache. My back ached all the time during my pregnancies, so I am not sure how this is different from one of those run-of-the-mill pregnancy complaints.

» A feeling of pressure, anywhere in your groin, pelvis or lower abdomen.

The second important development that happens with your baby around this time is that she can perceive light. The eyelids, which formerly were closed, are now able to open and the parts that make up the retina are now complete (44). Some people even say that if you shine a flashlight at your belly, your baby will put her hands up over her eyes. Your baby will also have be over 2.2 pounds (1000 grams) around this time. If you are having a boy, this is also approximately when the testes start to descend. For as many as a third of boys born preterm, and around four percent of boys born at term, the testes have not descended completely into the scrotum by the time they are born. In most instances, it will happen on its own by the time they are six months old.

Preterm Labour

It may seem early to be thinking about preterm labour, but if you are a mother who lost your last baby to preterm labour, you will be understandably nervous. Here are some statistics on preterm births in the United States that should give you a sense of the numbers: "Most preterm babies (71.2 percent) are born between 34 and 36 weeks of gestation. These are known as 'late' preterm births. Almost 13 percent of preterm babies are born between 32 and 33 weeks of gestation, about 10 percent between 28 and 31 weeks, and about 6 percent at less than 28 weeks." [63]. If your previous pregnancy was preterm, you face a slightly higher risk. While there are other risk factors that might increase the likelihood of preterm labour, often doctors do not know what caused it.

Only your doctor or midwife can tell for certain if what you are experiencing is preterm labour or false labour. They will check your cervix and monitor your contractions to see if they become stronger and more regular. However, some symptoms need to be checked right away. These are the ones listed in the urgent symptoms box.

Urgent Symptoms

» Bleeding
» Leaking fluid from your vagina (a sign your water has broken)
» Unusual, or constant, headaches (a sign your blood pressure is too high)
» Blurry vision or spots in your eyes (also a sign of high blood pressure)
» Dizziness
» Traumatic injury, like a fall or a motor vehicle accident [18]

Week 29

Welcome to your third trimester! You have made it through the first two and are into the final stretch. Some might say this is the hardest point, some would say the easiest. This is the point in pregnancy where most practitioners recommend you start to count kicks because they are now more regular and almost all women are able to feel them by this point. For many women with a loss, you have probably been counting them since the first movement you felt. In addition to the bracelet I mentioned in chapter six, kick-counter apps are another way to track fetal movement. If you have been using those methods informally as a way to keep your own anxieties at bay, now is the time to start being more methodical in your approach. You have made it this far!

Jenn decided not to formally count her kicks. As she described it, "they actually really discourage doing kick counts here (she is in the UK), maybe because it causes a lot of women to become overly worried or fixated. Our doctor here says know your body, know your baby, and trust your instincts. Every so often I think if I had not heard anything for a little while I probably could not pinpoint exactly how long it has been. I wait around or have a drink. As long as I feel something, I am okay." Charlotte also felt very ambivalent about kick counting. In her words: "The minute that kicks in, there's this degree of responsibility that seems to fall on you because before that point, you just have to trust and hope and keep your fingers crossed. But after 28 or 29 weeks, there's all this stuff like count the kicks and I found myself just getting more and more terrified. The whole concept, I just got terrified. I mean, she can have a quiet day, where she's moving, but just not as crazily, and then the anxiety.... You are in that grey zone where you know you are concerned, but should I be concerned or am I just paranoid? It's really difficult. They're supposed to have a pattern, and I do not know, maybe they do, but I am not 100 percent convinced. So I am not kick counting. Obviously I am aware of what she's doing, but I am not kick counting."

In the box below, I have added a review of some of the kick-counting apps available in the iTunes store at the time of writing this. You can either use these, or use the same criteria to evaluate the apps available on your device.

Kick-Counting Methods and Apps

Are you counting your kicks? Here in Canada, the Society of Obstetricians and Gynecologists of Canada recommends counting kicks starting at 26 weeks for women who have risk factors of a poor outcome.

In the UK, the Royal College of Obstetricians and Gynaecologists does not recommend specific kick counts, but does suggest that all women "be aware" of fetal movements [64]. Not every health care practitioner recommends it because there is some suggestion that it only adds anxiety without reducing the risk of stillbirth. However, if you are counting your kicks, either because your doctor recommends it or simply for your own anxiety, there are lots of apps available for your phone to help with kick counting. They are not all created equal, and they change all the time, so rather than recommend specific apps, here are some tips for how to choose the best app for your phone.

» Who developed this app? Was a medical professional (physician, midwife, other) involved in the design?

» How easy is it to use?

» Are there instructions? Are there links to support the methods used or did they use any research evidence?

» Are there any other features?

» What method of kick counting does it use?

Note: There are principally two methods. The Cardiff method asks you to count 10 movements and records how long it takes you to reach 10, usually within a 12-hour time frame. The Sandovsky method asks you to count a number of movements within a specific time frame (between 30 minutes and 2 hours).

9

WEEKS 30-36

Week 30

Week 30 marks the three-quarters mark. And with the likelihood that you will be early, this means you only have a couple more months to wait. Around this time, your baby will start producing their own blood cells in their bone marrow. This step increases the chances for survival outside the womb (60). This might be a good time to start considering whether you want to donate or bank your baby's cord blood. Depending on where you live, you can get a collection specimen from a private company to save your baby's cord blood for future use. At this time, there are limited uses for cord blood, and this option is expensive, although you may want to consider it as an insurance policy if your baby becomes sick with leukemia, which is one of the few diseases being treated with cord blood cells at this time. You can also consider donation, which would potentially provide this life-saving treatment to someone who has leukemia right now. It is particularly worth considering this option if you or your child are a member of a racial minority or are of mixed race. Just two days before my sons died, my sister received a bone marrow transplant from an anonymous donor. It was easy for her to find a donor because she, like her donor, was Caucasian. Sadly, there are fewer donors from minority populations, which makes it harder for people of colour or of mixed race to find a match. If you'd like to find out more about this option, in the United States you can contact **Be The Match** at **bethematch.org**. In Canada, contact **One Match** at **onematch.ca**.

Week 31

By week 31, your baby is starting to look very much like a full-term baby. There is still plenty of growing and weight gain that needs to take place. Your baby is about 11 inches (28 centimetres) long, and will weigh approximately four pounds (1800 grams) (14). If your baby were to be born today, their skin would still be very red and wrinkled, but otherwise would look pretty normal. Your baby will still have some of the protective hair (lanugo) on their torso, especially the shoulders and back, and they may still have this when they are born. They will be growing the hair on their heads too, at this point. One old wives' tale says that bad heartburn during pregnancy is a sign that you will have a hairy baby. I do not know if that is true or not—heartburn is stomach acid coming back up into your esophagus. Pregnancy makes it worse, both because of hormonal changes and because your stomach simply has less room due to the baby underneath. To relieve heartburn, you can try sitting or standing upright after meals, so you have more time to digest your food. You can try eating smaller meals more often, instead of the standard three meals a day. You can also try eating your food more slowly and chewing more carefully. Some other suggestions for managing heartburn include not drinking fluids during your meals and avoiding gas-producing foods or things that are overly spicy or greasy. If you are still bothered by heartburn, talk to your doctor or pharmacist before taking any over-the-counter medications. These medications can become less effective over time and can interfere with your body's ability to absorb other medications you might be taking.

Baby Showers and Blessingways

When you are pregnant for the second time or third time or more, you might not feel comfortable with a baby shower. Depending on your cultural traditions, baby showers may not even be something you have considered. Some people will not have a baby shower before the baby is born because of a superstitious feeling that they are bad luck. With my first pregnancy I had two baby showers, one thrown by a dear friend, the other by my coworkers. While I have a lot of wonderful memories of both of these occasions, after Nate and Sam died, the showers wracked me with guilt. We had a room full of unopened presents and I felt terrible knowing that so many people had been generous with their time and money, only to have no baby to show for it. I was torn about whether I should give the gifts back, whether I should store them for another baby, or whether I should give them away. With my subsequent pregnancies I wanted nothing to do with baby showers. My friends from my book club decided to have a surprise shower for me—it was very small, and the only gifts given were books. For me, it was perfect. If you feel uncomfortable about the thought of a baby shower, you might want to consider an alternative: a Blessingway. The word Blessingway comes from a Navajo tradition, which provides a spiritual rite of passage to a pregnant woman and protects her from the complications of pregnancy.

What is a Blessingway? According to one book on the subject, "Blessingways are woman-centered celebrations. The emphasis in a Blessingway ceremony is on heralding the expectant mother—her strength, her beauty, her dignity, her womanhood, her divine procreative powers, her metamorphosis as she goes through the creative process of bringing new life into this world" (65). And if that seems a little too new-agey for your taste, here's another definition: "A Blessingway is about the mother and the birth process. We are going to weave a web of protection and love and honor and respect around this woman. We are not gathering to deal with the baby; this is all about the mother" (65). In that definition, I really like the idea of the Blessingway as an alternative to a baby shower. It takes the focus off the baby and what gifts the baby might need, and instead puts the emphasis on the mother. Instead of all the "stuff," it focuses on what you need as a mother to prepare yourself for the upcoming birth and the changes it will bring to your life. As someone who has previously had a child, or several children, you may feel that you already have all the things you need. You have a crib and a change table and onesies and toys. Or, you may simply feel that it is still too premature to celebrate this new life. But if you have friends and family who are excited about your pregnancy and want to have a celebration, this may be a good compromise. Because a Blessingway is more about the mother, you can make the gifts more ceremonial than material. Here are just a few ideas of activities you can plan for a Blessingway.

Body Painting and Henna Tattoos

Ingredients For Henna Paste

» Henna powder (one ounce will decorate about 12 hands, or enough for six people)

» A small amount of very strong tea or coffee. This should still be hot!

» Two lemons or limes

» A tea strainer or a fine sieve

» A wooden or stainless steel spoon

» A ceramic, glass or stainless steel bowl to mix the henna

» A small bowl for the lemon or lime juice

A general rule in mixing henna is that the more acidic the mixture, the darker the stain. If the paste does not give a dark enough stain, add lemon or lime juice to the paste.

Steps

1. Using a strainer, sift henna powder into a bowl.

2. Strain the juice from a lemon or lime into the bowl and stir with the henna powder. Add enough lemon or lime juice so that the henna powder becomes a thick paste.

3. Add a small amount of very hot, strong tea or coffee and stir so that it becomes a thick paste, about the consistency of toothpaste. Cover the henna paste and leave it overnight for the dye to develop.

*Recipe adapted from **hennamehndi.com***

Body painting and henna tattooing are two fun options for celebrating your round belly...if you are comfortable showing it off in front of friends and family! Henna tattoos will last longer, possibly even until you give birth. Both options allow you to sit back and enjoy being pampered while your friends take their time attending to your needs. They fit perfectly with the spirit of a Blessingway. If you have never had a henna tattoo before, you do not need to draw freehand—there are lots of stencils available online to help you with the designs.

Body painting provides you with a more colourful, but temporary, option. You might need to be a bit of a better artist for this option, but if you have the skills it can be quite beautiful. You can have everyone who attends your Blessingway "sign" your belly with their wishes for this baby. You can also find all kinds of beautiful ideas on Pinterest.

Friendship Necklace

This is another great idea for a Blessingway, as it allows friends and family who live far away to participate. Ask everyone to send a bead representing each of their pregnancies (this works well if you have a lot of friends you have met through the online baby loss community). At your Blessingway, string the beads together to make a large necklace that you can wear until the baby is born. Each bead represents the collective strength of the women who have gone through this transition before you. I found it amazing to see how many of my friends included beads for their miscarriages as well as the babies who were born, so it can be a powerful reminder than you are not alone. Also, because everyone has chosen their own beads, your necklace will be a little eclectic and definitely one of a kind!

Candle Lighting

A candle-lighting ceremony can be a peaceful way to acknowledge both the past and the future. Buy enough large pillar candles for everyone who will be attending your Blessingway. Have everyone stand in a circle and dim the lights. As the pregnant mother, you can go around the circle and light each person's candle, and as you do so, have them say something they admire about you or a quality you have that makes you a good mother. Once all the candles are lit, you can sit in the silence for a moment and treasure the positive thoughts your friends and family have shared. Ask your friends to each take the candle home with them to keep. When they hear your labour has started, they can light their candles in solidarity with you and leave it lit until they hear the good news that your baby has arrived safely.

Freezer Potluck

Instead of gifts, ask everyone to bring a dish that can easily be popped in the freezer for later. This will provide you with some fabulous ready-made meals for when you are time-starved. In those first few days after baby is born, this can be a much better gift than another Diaper Genie!

There are tons of great Blessingway ideas available, but the key to remember is that this is meant as a more intimate, spiritual gathering that is focused on the mother. You can still have many of the baby shower games, or gifts, if you feel comfortable with them, but you should be at the centre. Some other ideas for mom-centred gifts include a pregnancy photography session with a professional photographer (find one at Now I Lay Me Down to Sleep (NowILayMeDowntoSleep.org)—let them know you support their volunteer work with the organization!); a pregnancy massage; a nice pair of pyjamas, dressing gown and slippers, for those days you just do not have the energy to get dressed; an offer to look after older children when the baby gets here, etc.

Maeve had a Blessingway for her pregnancy after loss. She described how important the experience was for her: "We had more than 40 people here. It was a big day. I mostly organized it. I think you are meant to have a girlfriend organize it for you, but no one offered, so I just organized it myself. It was really emotional. We had lots of tears and lots of talking about Cord. That was really wonderful. People do not know how to be there for you. When you have something that people can celebrate, they come out in droves and are really happy to support us. I wish they had been there during the other time. But I accept that it is not easy to know how to be there. All of the beautiful things that people were saying and what they think about Cord and all this sort of stuff. But we had such a lovely day. We had a really nice day and everyone came and everyone had a really good time."

Buying things for the new baby can feel good or can come with mixed emotions. Regina certainly felt torn. She describes it as being "so exciting, because I can go into a baby store again. Before I totally avoided it. When I went to a store and they have a baby section I would turn before I could get there. I couldn't see anything. But now, I get to go and it's so nice, but at the same time, all those memories come back. It's happy and it's sad at the same time." She was around 20 weeks when she started to feel comfortable buying things for the new baby.

As Regina says, "it is weird for me to see baby stuff around the house. When we lost Jacob, we didn't touch anything from his bedroom for two months, and then I put his things, like the crib and his toys and clothes…I just put it away. So I just bought a few things for her, because it's hard not to. It makes it real, getting things for her. Before you didn't want to think about buying anything because you are just so terrified. But she's here. I know she's here. She's moving and everything. So I have to. In the same way I did it for Jacob, I have to do it for her. I want to."

Week 32

By week 32, your baby is continuing to gain weight and getting ready to be born. Your baby will still be making vigorous kicks despite the fact that they are running out of room, so you will want to continue to measure movement and let your doctor know about any decrease. There will be rolls, flutters, baby hiccups, and other movements, so you should be feeling things happening. Remember, if you have concerns, the doctors and nurses are there for you and you should never feel embarrassed about calling them, asking for extra appointments, or doing whatever it takes for you to feel reassured.

Particularly because you have made it so close to the end, they should be eager to help see you through this final hurdle of the last few weeks. Some of the things they will be looking for at your checkups will depend on whether you were given a diagnosis during this pregnancy or a cause of death during your last. The more frequent ultrasounds will measure things like the quantity of amniotic fluid and signs of preeclampsia. Preeclampsia is a type of high blood pressure that happens during pregnancy. Even if you have never had high blood pressure before, you can be at risk of this condition, which affects between five and ten percent of all pregnant women (18). Some of the symptoms you might experience include headaches or swelling, pain or discomfort, or changes to your vision. To test for this, the nurse will check your blood pressure at every visit and may also check for protein in your urine. If you develop preeclampsia at this late stage in your pregnancy, you will likely be induced. The only cure for preeclampsia is delivery of the baby.

Week 33

In addition to weight gain, these last few weeks of pregnancy are important for developing the baby's lungs. Even though the baby still gets all the oxygen they need through the umbilical cord, the lungs are growing and developing right up until delivery. The respiratory muscles develop much earlier, and movements of the chest wall can be seen on ultrasounds as early as 11 weeks. Your doctor has been checking for practice-breathing movements on ultrasounds, and these movements are helping to move amniotic fluid through the respiratory tract (14). However, your baby's lungs are still developing their ability to produce surfactant, which is a liquid-like substance that helps keep your lungs open when you breathe. In some cases, your doctor may give you corticosteroids, which can encourage the development of surfactant. This may be the case when a preterm birth is expected.

Week 34

In addition to your baby's lungs developing, the brain is also growing. As much as one-third of a baby's brain size develops in the last few weeks of pregnancy. This is one reason your health care provider may want you to wait as long as possible before delivering your baby. Yet if you do go into labour this early, rest assured that your child will more than likely be healthy, happy, and intellectually at their fullest capacity. Babies born at 34 weeks are considered late-preterm, and make up over 70 percent of all babies born preterm (63). Particularly if you had an early labour last time, you will want to watch carefully for symptoms of preterm labour, mentioned in chapter eight. During these last couple of weeks before delivery, your baby will also continue to gain weight and become stronger.

Week 35

By this point, your baby may also be in the head-down position, getting ready to be born. It may feel by this stage that your baby is running out of room. However, if your baby is breech, she may still turn before delivery. Babies still find a way to move around, even this late in the pregnancy. With my daughter, she seemed to like gymnastics, regularly changing her position.

What is Moxibustion?

According to Natural Standard, moxibustion is "a therapeutic method in traditional Chinese medicine, classical (five element) acupuncture, and Japanese acupuncture in which an herb, usually mugwort (Artemisia vulgaris), is burned above the skin or on the acupuncture points for the purpose of introducing heat into an acupuncture point to alleviate symptoms." (15)

Moxibustion, which is a form of traditional Chinese medicine often used in conjunction with acupuncture, has been used historically to correct a breech baby and encourage them to turn downwards. I decided to try it. When I went in to hospital to have my labour induced, sure enough she had turned head down. The next morning, when it was time to actually start labour, she was back in a breech position, so I am not entirely sure it worked. I ended up having an external cephalic version despite the moxibustion.

Since my daughter's birth, more studies have been done into the use of moxibustion to prevent breech presentation and the results are fairly limited. While there is some suggestion that moxibustion combined with acupuncture or postural exercises may reduce the need for cesarean sections and breech presentations at birth, the studies were not of the highest quality [66]. Moxibustion may work for you, or like me, it may not.

External Cephalic Version

An external cephalic version is a procedure in which a doctor (or sometimes two) uses pressure from the outside to manually rotate your baby into the correct position. In can be done well before you give birth, at around 36 to 37 weeks, or even while you are in labour, as long as your waters have not yet broken [67]. While a nurse keeps the ultrasound on your baby to monitor their position and heart rate, the doctor will place their hands on your stomach, right on the baby's head and rear. They will then manually turn them around. It is usually only done if you have had a baby before at term and if you have not had a previous cesarean section. It does hurt, so you may be given medication for the pain. As with all medical procedures, there are risks, so they will not do it if your baby shows signs of distress, if you have certain medical conditions, or if there are other reasons to suggest you might need a cesarean section. I had an external cephalic version done in my fourth pregnancy with my daughter, the morning I was induced. The resident and attending physician worked together while a nurse monitored on the ultrasound. Because my daughter had previously been head down, I had never had a cesarean birth and my previous term pregnancy was twins, they knew that I would likely be a good candidate for this procedure. This time, she stayed in the right position.

Week 36

Week 36 is the last week of preterm, so your body is really preparing itself for birth now. If you still have not made preparations, like buying a car seat, do not worry. My husband and I found this to be one of the most stressful preparations we made, because we were terrified of spending any money or buying anything new until the baby arrived. While mothers are spending a lot less time in hospital than they did in their parents' generation, with some mothers choosing to go home the same day, you will still likely have lots of time to make this purchase even if you wait until the baby is here! This can definitely be a task for a grandparent to keep them occupied during labour.

Unless you are at risk for a preterm birth, this will likely be when your doctor or midwife will order a strep B test. Group B streptococcus are common bacteria that can be treated with antibiotics. While mostly harmless for mothers, who might never know they have it, group B streptococcus can be serious if the baby becomes infected during the delivery process. The most common way for testing for the presence of these bacteria is to use a cotton swab to swab your vagina [18]. Your doctor will likely ask you to do this yourself while you are there for your regular visit. The lab will then take the swab to see if the bacteria grow. Another way of testing for group B streptococcus is by taking a urine sample. If you test positive for the bacteria, meaning they find it present in your urine or on the swab, you will be given antibiotics during labour. You may also be given these antibiotics as a precaution if you go into labour before they have a chance to test you and if you are in a high-risk category, such as having had a previous group B streptococcus infection, if you have an unexplained fever, or if your water breaks more than 18 hours before labour begins.

10

WEEKS 37-40

Week 37

A big congratulations for making it this far. After week 37, your baby is considered to be full term, which is the healthiest time —both for you and your baby—to be born. Even if your baby is not here yet, you can think of this moment as a big milestone. In this chapter you'll find information about different ways women who have had a loss have given birth in their next pregnancy. Whatever you decide, together with your health care provider, please know that there is no right or wrong answer. Whatever you choose, you will need to take into consideration your own personal circumstances, your physical and mental health, as well as the health of your baby. You will also want to consider your own level of comfort with risks and the expertise and training of the doctors, midwives or nurses you will be working with. No matter what, you will be making trade-offs and trying to find the best balance for your own physical and mental health needs. Take the time to consider all options, listen carefully to the advice of your doctor or midwife, and know that whatever happens, you are making the right choice.

Maeve talks about her anxiety over choosing whether or not to be induced and how talking it over with another mother who had experienced a pregnancy after a loss was helpful.

In Maeve's words

I am scared about the birth. Having Shelli to talk to about it helped a lot because she has had live babies. When I gave birth to Cord, it was just Gavin and I and the midwife. I know that it will be quite different with this baby. They treat you differently. I started to not be that happy about being induced, but then I started to think that I just cannot go into labour naturally. I will be really stressed! We live more than half an hour away (from the hospital). What if she comes quickly? So we suddenly felt trapped: damned if I do, damned if I did not. But Shelli said to me, 'Remember, you had a really good birth with Cord. This baby will be alive and it will help you when you are giving birth. This baby is going to want to come out. It is going to want to help you.' That just made so much difference to me.

Jenn describes her own fear about the birth. "My biggest worry is that it is going to happen again. I don't feel confident at all that we are going to bring our baby home. I don't know that we will until I walk through the door with one. But I also worry about how I will feel physically to not be pregnant anymore." She continued to say this time she is trying "to throw that away and let myself imagine what it will be like, and let myself plan, and think about things in more detail. In some ways that has really helped. It has given me a positive focus."

Giving Birth: Induction

Choosing to induce labour before 40 weeks is the most popular decision for moms who have had a previous loss, especially if this loss was at term and unexplained (68). This does not mean it is what you will want, or that you will be eligible for this option, but do know that you are not alone in feeling uncomfortable, both emotionally and physically, waiting for the whole 40 weeks. Reading much of the traditional pregnancy literature might make you fearful of induction before term. Campaigns by the Association of Women's Health, Obstetric and Neonatal Nurses, and the American College of Obstetricians and Gynecologists (ACOG) encourage women to wait the full 40 weeks. However, even in their literature, they emphasize that there are medical reasons to have an induction, such as high blood pressure (69). Your mental health and anxiety level should be taken into consideration and psychosocial reasons are considered appropriate by the ACOG (14). Remember, their information campaign is targeting first-time moms, so many of the risks are lower for you if your first pregnancy was induced after no heartbeat was found. If you already know your body is capable of handling an induced labour, then this option may be right for you. In the United States, approximately three percent of births are induced before 39 weeks for "non-medical reasons," which is a very narrowly defined list (70).

With an induction, your doctor will take several steps to encourage labour to happen. Which methods she uses, or how much, will depend on your personal circumstances and hospital policy. Often, the first step is to ripen your cervix by using a gel or suppository. This medicine contains the hormone prostaglandin and works to soften your cervix and help it get ready for delivering your baby. Another method of ripening the cervix is to use laminaria, which is actually dried kelp. Sometimes a small balloon-like catheter can be inserted, to help make the cervix wider. If your cervix is already ripe, your doctor might skip this step altogether.

The next step might be to rupture the membranes, also called breaking your waters, if it does not happen on its own. This is done by using a small device that looks a little like a crochet hook. It can be a little uncomfortable, but not painful.

Last, a drug called oxytocin can be given to bring on your contractions. Oxytocin is a hormone that is naturally produced by your body when you are in labour. This drug also has a use in augmentation: it's given to women who have gone into labour naturally but who need help to speed things up. The development of synthetic oxytocin is so wonderful, Vincent du Vigneaud won the Nobel Prize for discovering how to produce it (14). Before it was available, women were given oxytocin that came from pigs.

There is absolutely no difference between the oxytocin you produce yourself and the oxytocin produced synthetically. They are identical chemical structures. The drug is given intravenously and is sometimes called by the brand name Pitocin. When you are given oxytocin, either for a labour induction or a labour augmentation, you will need to be monitored closely because the amount a woman needs varies widely. Nurses will use two external devices, one to monitor your contractions, the other to monitor your baby's heartbeat. Usually, you will be started on a very low dose, and the dose will be increased as needed, roughly every 15-40 minutes.

While risks associated with induction are low, there are some instances where having an induced labour is not recommended. Examples of this might be if your baby is considered too large for a vaginal delivery, a condition called macrosomia, or if you have some uterine scarring from previous surgeries, including previous cesarean sections. If you can wait for labour to happen naturally, you will also lower your risks of the baby having jaundice, or having respiratory problems and needing a stay in the Neonatal Intensive Care Unit (NICU). Talk to your doctor about which option is right for you and whether there are ways you can manage your anxiety.

Charlotte chose to be induced and jokes that she never would have considered it for her first pregnancy. "With my first pregnancy, I thought that induction was the devil's work, you know, this is what I was learning! About the cascading interventions, and how it will all end up in a cesarean, you know, the worst case scenario! Oh no! Whereas now, the question is not if I will be induced, it is when. At 37 weeks? Or can I hang in with the hope that, I could be a real strong trailblazer and hold off."

Steph also chose to be induced, and describes it as a trust exercise. She had to learn to trust both her own body and her doctor, a woman with plenty of experience in delivering babies through induction. In Steph's words: "I have a general idea of what is going to happen and what I want to happen. It still makes me nervous because I have no control over it. I am just going and letting things progress and doing what my doctor thinks is the best course of action and trusting that she has done it once before. Putting all that trust into someone else makes me nervous, but that is what I have to do." She describes how she couldn't just wait for things to happen, because "the anxiety and the fear are too much. I have to be where the doctors are, I have to be where what needs to be done can be done."

Week 38

By week 38, your baby is considered term and ready to arrive very soon. While the baby continues to grow, your weight increase should be stopping by now. Because your baby has been swallowing amniotic fluid, the first bowel movement, called meconium, is forming in the intestines. Meconium is "made up of salts, amniotic fluid, mucus, bile, and epithelial (skin) cells. This substance is greenish black, almost odorless, and tarry" (71). Interestingly, the word meconium comes from the Greek word for poppies, probably because someone thought it looked like poppy juice or poppy seeds. If your baby expels this meconium before being born, the amniotic fluid can look dark, a condition called meconium staining. This happens in about 20 percent of babies born at term (14).

When this happens, your baby can be at risk for breathing in the substance when they are first born. This can lead to a condition called meconium aspiration syndrome, something that happens in less than two percent of births. Breathing in meconium can cause damage to the lungs and may require some serious interventions. Even if the meconium has been expelled before birth, the risk can be reduced by cleaning and suctioning baby's nose and mouth before they are fully born and then further tracheal suctioning after birth to try and remove as much meconium as possible before baby takes her first breath. It cannot be prevented before birth, but some risk factors that make meconium staining, and therefore meconium aspiration, more likely, include preeclampsia, hypertension, fetal growth restriction, and being overdue (71).

Giving Birth: Scheduled Cesarean Birth

Another option when giving birth is to have a scheduled cesarean section. This option is more likely if your last baby was delivered by cesarean section, especially if it was recently. You may also be offered a cesarean if your baby is in a breech position and cannot be turned using an external cephalic version, or there are other medical reasons to suggest that this option might be best for you and your baby. Many people, including ACOG, are concerned about the rise in cesarean deliveries, as rates in the United States have been increasing. Cesarean rates reached as high as 30 percent of births in 2007, when the US Department of Health and Human Services, together with ACOG, launched a goal to reduce cesareans to just 15 percent of births (14). There are some good reasons for this concern, as cesarean births do have a higher rate of complications—despite being low risk, it is still serious surgery. However, if, after consulting with your doctor, you decide that a cesarean birth is your best option, then there is nothing to feel guilty about. You are not missing out on an important experience (which is seriously overrated), or recklessly endangering your health. Only you and your doctor know your personal circumstances. Together you can make the best choice for your unique situation.

With a cesarean section, the nurse will prepare your belly by washing it to reduce the likelihood of infection. You will also have a catheter put in to drain your urine because, with an anesthetic, you will not be able to feel your bladder. You will also be given an IV to administer the anesthetic, which is usually a regional anesthetic (sometimes called a spinal block or epidural). This will allow you to be awake during the entire procedure. In some instances, you might need a general anesthetic, which means you will be asleep. The regional anesthetic will completely numb you from the breasts down.

Once you are safely anesthetized and unable to feel anything, the doctor will make a small incision, just above your pubic bone. This is called a bikini cut. The doctor will cut the uterus open next, usually horizontally (from left to right across your belly), but sometimes vertically (up and down from your public area to your stomach). This is decided based on what position your baby is in, but if you have had a previous cesarean birth, the scarring from that operation will be taken into consideration. The third layer is the amniotic sac, and the doctor will cut this next to take your baby out. The umbilical cord will be cut and your placenta will be removed. Then the doctor will close the incisions he made with either medical staples or stitches. Due to the anesthetic, you should not feel pain during this procedure, but you will feel pushing, prodding, or tugging as these steps are taken.

Full recovery from a cesarean birth takes about four to six weeks. You will likely need to stay in hospital longer than if you gave birth vaginally, usually about three days. You can breastfeed immediately after a cesarean birth and should get up to walk around as soon as you can manage. Ask the nurse, personal support worker, or physiotherapist assigned to you to help you get up and walk for the first few times, because the anesthetic will make you wobbly and likely to fall at first. One of the most common complications from a cesarean birth is an infection, so you need to keep an eye out for fever, pain, or redness at your incision site. Be sure to follow instructions on post-partum care. If you need more information about planning for a cesarean birth, there are some great resources, including videos, at **http://www. nlm.nih.gov/medlineplus/cesareansection.html**.

Because Jenn lost Fiona during labour, she opted for a scheduled cesarean birth. For her, this was the best option. As she described it: "Having a team around you that consistently acknowledges what you have been through was really important for me because Fiona wasn't forgotten at all along the way. Every appointment we had, she was mentioned at some point. I think for me that is what made all the difference. Having things as planned and predictable as possible for me was really important. I think particularly because of the loss happening during labour. To take that risk of spontaneous labour away even as a possibility this time around was important to me, although it never completely gets rid of the worry. Eliminating as much of the unpredictability as possible was helpful to me, so knowing well in advance when I was going in, and what time it was going to be and who was going to be there. All those things."

Weeks 39–40

You are so close now! By week 39, your baby is only growing at a slow pace, but there are still changes happening. The lanugo hair that kept her warm in the uterus is starting to disappear. Also, vernix, the waxy, cheesy substance preterm babies have, is starting to disappear too. If your baby were born now, they might have very little of it left.

Giving Birth: Waiting for Labour to Start on Its Own

If you have decided to wait for labour to start on its own, congratulations. You are one brave momma! While waiting for labour to start naturally can seem like a given for most mothers, for those of us pregnant after a loss it is the least-chosen option. Whether you were induced last time or had a cesarean birth or went into labour naturally, waiting for labour to start is usually the healthiest option for both you and baby. It reduces the likelihood of your baby needing extra care in the NICU due to jaundice or respiratory issues. It has a much shorter recovery time than a cesarean birth. But you will need to consider your own circumstances before deciding if this is right for you.

If you did not go into labour naturally before, I can let you in on a secret: Labour is not exactly as you see on television. Popular media likes to show a woman waking up to a puddle in her bed (her waters breaking), her husband frantically getting to the car and helping her downstairs (while contractions that she mysteriously did not feel two minutes ago make it hard for her to walk), and the baby being delivered at the side of the road by a taxi driver and a paramedic. Most of the time it is agonizingly slow. There are principally three early signs that you might experience, and you may not even notice all of them.

The first is called bloody show, which is an awful name and I wish someone would come up with a better one. It is not actually a medical term, but a way of describing how, when your cervix dilates to get ready to go into labour, the small amount of mucus that was plugging the cervix comes loose. It can cause a thick, mucussy discharge to come out of your vagina (this is the "show")(18). Because your cervix is softening and widening, there can be a tiny amount of blood in the show, which might make it appear a little pink (this is the bloody part). Or not. Sometimes this mucussy discharge is clear. Or, it might have happened and you did not notice. Coming up with a better name for this would be helpful because I know I imagined a giant cork, or bathtub plug, covered in blood and popping out in the toilet. This can happen several days before labour begins, so seeing your bloody show does not mean you need to leap into the car and rush to the hospital just yet. However, you might want to call your doctor just to let them know. And if there are significant amounts of blood, be sure to go to hospital right away.

The second sign is having your water break. This is also often nothing like they show on television, where it usually takes place in your bed or at the supermarket, looks a lot like Niagara Falls, and also means that the baby is seconds away from popping out. In reality, when your waters break (also called ruptured membranes), it can be a small leak or a more dramatic gush. Usually your water is pale coloured, not clear, although it could also be darker and a brownish colour if there is meconium staining. Having your waters break is a more reliable indicator that labour is about to begin than the bloody show, but it usually does not mean labour will happen immediately. You should still go to hospital. Many women need to have their waters broken after contractions have already begun, so do not be surprised if your water never breaks on its own.

The third sign that labour is beginning are contractions. If you have experienced Braxton-Hicks contractions at any point in your pregnancy, then these will feel very similar but will be increasing in frequency and intensity. Contractions are just a contracting of the uterus (hence the name), so it will feel as though your uterus will tighten and then loosen up again without you being able to control it (18). Contractions are short, lasting less than a minute, although they can certainly feel like an eternity when you are having one. It is possible to have painless contractions, and some women do not feel anything until they are well into the second phase of labour, also called the active phase. If you are experiencing contractions that are regular, even if they are not yet five minutes apart, go to the hospital.

Labour

Whether you are induced or go into labour on your own, the stages of labour are very similar. Even women who go into labour naturally may have it "augmented" with labour induction techniques, such as a manual rupture of the membranes or the use of oxytocin.

There are essentially three stages of labour. The first, which is what most of us think of as labour, is where you get contractions and dilated cervix. In the second stage you are fully dilated and are told to start pushing. This lasts until your baby is born. The third stage is from the time baby is born until the placenta is delivered (18).

To further complicate things, the first stage is subdivided into three phases. In the first phase, sometimes called the latent phase, your cervix is just starting to dilate. In the active phase dilation grows from one to three inches (three to eight centimetres). The transition phase happens when the cervix dilates the last inch. There is no set time for each of these three phases to happen, and the changes in the first phase are often so small many women don't even know they are in labour.

Depending on the circumstances of your last birth, labour may be a time when you are very anxious. In my case, I felt more relaxed at this point than I had during the entire pregnancy because I finally felt like this baby was going to arrive safely. I spent more time trying to manage my husband's anxiety than I did mine! Every time the fetal monitor slipped a little bit, he would push the call button to get the nurse. If your last labour was very stressful, you will want to have several ways to keep your anxiety in check. Being relaxed during birth can make things easier. Some options you might consider include breathing techniques, hypnotherapy, or hydrotherapy (either a shower or a tub). In the early phases of labour, simply bringing a good book to read, watching television, or playing games on your phone may be all you need to distract you.

As labour progresses, you may want medication to reduce the pain. As far as I am concerned, a woman who has lost a baby is already a martyr to the baby cause, so why suffer more than you have to? If the question is drugs, the answer is yes! However, I fully recognize that this is not right for everyone. The most common pain relief used in labour is an epidural. Another option is nitrous oxide, or laughing gas. It is not common in the United States, but is regularly used in other countries and provides a milder pain relief.

Once the baby is out, you will have two choices: to have the baby placed on your chest immediately, or to have baby checked and weighed first. If there are any complications, of course, the neonatal team may have to swoop in anyway. For several reasons, many professionals will advocate for placing baby on your chest right away. I actually chose the other option because I was nervous and wanted them to be sure everything was okay before I saw my daughter. It only took a couple minutes, and I was busy delivering the placenta. I remain convinced that my daughter will not grow up to be deprived as a result of this short interval away from me.

Once that baby is on your chest, you will probably feel relieved, excited, exhausted and thrilled to meet your new little one. After all the anxiety, stress, and work of the past few years, you have what you have always wanted. A precious little baby. Take lots of pictures, this moment is beautiful.

11

BABY'S HERE

When your new baby comes, some people will act as though you can now forget the baby you have lost. However, while you may be writing a whole new chapter in your life, you are not erasing the chapters that came before it. You will still miss your baby who died. Being a mother to a living child has challenges enough, but you will be influenced by your experience in having a baby who did not survive. Because you may have held back emotionally during your pregnancy, a little part of you may have been afraid that this baby would not be born alive. Some researchers have found that women who have had a pregnancy loss are somewhat emotionally numb when their living baby is first born (72). Feel free to take this "getting to know you" stage slowly. You may find that your fears are heightened, so that normal changes in the baby seem much more concerning.

This is common, and you may need additional reassurance from your nurses and doctors that everything is okay. When my daughter was born, she was taken to the NICU with concerns over jaundice and her weight gain. The nurses encouraged me to get a couple hours sleep and they would wake me when it came time to feed her. After no more than an hour, I woke with a nightmare. The fear of my baby being taken from me was just too overwhelming. The nurse took me to my daughter so that I could see her and be reassured that everything was fine. Having the nurse show me not just that she was okay, but providing me with specifics on why they knew she was going to be okay, helped. With each bit of encouragement I received—that I would be able to bring her home soon, that I could continue to breastfeed, that I would have support when I got home too—I gained confidence in my abilities as a mom.

Breastfeeding

Breastfeeding can be one of the healthiest and most beautiful ways to bond with your baby, but that does not mean it is always easy. Because your last baby died, you may still be struggling with feelings that you failed as a mother in protecting your child. Those emotions can spill over into breastfeeding (72). I want to reassure you that you did not fail as a mother and that you can successfully breastfeed. Breastfeeding is how most babies are fed, at least initially, and it is healthiest for both baby and mother. In most cases, you can still breastfeed if you are taking medication (ask your doctor, pharmacist, or nurse for advice regarding the specific medications you are taking). While breastfeeding may be the most common and natural way to feed a baby, it can be hard. There will be times when you feel frustrated or disappointed in breastfeeding, but you can stick with it.

If you find you need extra support, here are some suggestions for how and where to find it:

»   If you decided to skip prenatal classes, you may have missed out on a group of mothers who are going through the same struggles as you. Consider contacting your public health nurse to see if there are mother support groups for breastfeeding in your area.

»   La Leche League is an international organization that is dedicated to supporting breastfeeding mothers. They have a variety of programs depending on where you live, but often offer both group and one-on-one support, and a telephone hotline.

»   Many nurses and midwives are also International Board Certified Lactation Consultants (IBCLC). This means that they have additional education in teaching women how to breastfeed effectively, and how to support women who are having trouble. IBCLCs work in a variety of settings: private practice, hospitals, public health units, midwifery offices, and more. Look on their website to find one near you: **www.ilca.org**.

At first, Jenn had trouble breastfeeding. She describes how hard it was: "We had trouble with breastfeeding for the first two and a half weeks. I was expressing and feeding her with a bottle, and that was a huge difficulty. That feeling that this is not how it is supposed to be, but because she was so little she struggled to latch. I found it really tough because we were in the hospital and I felt quite manhandled all of the time by all of the midwives. They were very supportive and hands-on, but it was really difficult because Evelyn wasn't able to do it and I couldn't figure out why. When I got home, it was good to be home. I can do this the way that I wanted to do this. It was more relaxed." Jenn was able to get Evelyn latching correctly and breastfeeding successfully at that point.

I also struggled with my daughter Rebecca. At first, my husband and I tracked every feed to the minute, terrified she would not be getting enough. As the weeks passed and I gained confidence in my ability to feed her, this became less necessary for us. She was gaining weight. She was happy. I spent more time listening to the lactation consultants and my doctor's advice and less time listening to my own negative talk.

If you choose to formula feed, or have to for health reasons, this does not mean you failed. Many women use formula to feed their babies, for a variety of reasons. Breastfeeding may not be right for you or your baby. Do what you need to do to feel healthy, both physically and emotionally.

Renewed Grief and Postpartum Depression

Depression is one of the most common mental health issues, and postpartum depression is common. An estimated 11 percent of women experience depression during pregnancy and 14 percent of women experience postpartum depression [73]. There are factors that can make experiencing depression after baby is born more likely, such as not having a lot of support from your family, being an older or younger than average mom, or having a history of depression. Having lost a baby is another factor that increases your risk. In one study, more than half of the women who lost a child met the criteria for depression in the year after the birth of a live baby [74]. One-third of them experienced anxiety. Also, the more losses a woman had, the more likely she was to experience depression.

Whether this is the old pre-baby depression coming back or a new incidence of postpartum depression may be splitting hairs. The important thing to remember is that you are not alone in feeling this way. There is help available. When I was depressed after my daughter was born, I felt guilty because I did not think I deserved to feel this way. The one thing that I had ached for, yearned for, and hoped for over the past three years was finally here. I had thought my sadness would vanish as soon as my baby arrived. I was shocked when it did not. I did not think I had any right to feel sad. My daughter was happy and healthy. Unfortunately, that is how the twisted thinking of depression works. I was mistaken in thinking that having a baby would be a magic cure for my loss. Having a newborn is hard work, and it remains hard work even if you have had a loss. The hormonal changes that make depression more likely in the postpartum period still happen if you have had a pregnancy loss. And of course, as much as you love your living baby, you did not stop loving and missing the baby you lost. Seeing your healthy child go through their developmental milestones can just be a sad reminder of what you missed (and will continue to miss) with their brother or sister.

If, at any point, you are concerned about yourself or your partner, please ask for help. There is no need to continue to suffer alone, and there are therapies available that can help. I was very lucky to have the support of a mother's group for women who have postpartum depression. In a small group led by a social worker, we talked through our issues and it helped to feel less alone. If you need medication to help get you through this period, your doctor can help you find the right one. You can take most antidepressants safely while breastfeeding, and your doctor and pharmacist will advise you on this (75). If you were seeing a therapist before your baby was born, you may find it helpful to go back to them, even if only for a few sessions. They can help gauge your risk, work with you to find coping strategies and refer you to additional help if needed. If you find yourself overwhelmed, place your baby in a safe space and take a few minutes to calm yourself down. A few times, I had to put my daughter in her crib, then I would go into the bathroom and turn on the hairdryer just to drown out the sound of the crying! If you need more time, call a friend or a family member to babysit, or even put the baby in a stroller and go for a walk. It is okay to ask for help and you are not alone in needing help to get through this challenging time.

Learning to Bond with This Baby

There is some indication that having a stillbirth or early neonatal death can make bonding with your new baby a challenge. You may have spent a lot of time and energy during your pregnancy protecting your heart. You may have fears that your lost child will be forgotten now that your other baby is here, and certainly that might be the message you have been receiving from well-meaning friends and relatives. Now that the baby is here, you will want to develop a strong bond and consider different ways to achieve that.

Some researchers have concerns that when a baby is born after a loss, the mother will idealize their deceased child. In their minds, the baby who died was a perfect angel, while the baby in front of them is very much a real human, with all their faults and imperfections. As one researcher described it, "mothers with a history of loss continued to view their infants as being less ideal than did the group of women without a history of loss" (76). However, even if you view your baby as less than ideal, it does not mean you are not forming a loving, healthy bond. Much of the research on "replacement child" syndrome was done on older children anyway (76).

Another way your parenting may have changed is that you have become overprotective of this baby. Knowing all the things that could possibly go wrong, you may find yourself frequently checking when the baby is sleeping to be sure that they are still breathing, or double- and triple-checking the car seat to be certain they are strapped in just right (77). In one example of my own paranoia, while riding a (15-minute!) ferry I took my daughter out of her car seat and held her in my lap because I was terrified that the boat might sink and I would not be able to get her out of her car seat in time. Acknowledging that you are having these fears, that you recognize that they are not rational, and that you need to take certain steps to feel that you and your baby are safe, can help you feel better about your fears and about your abilities as a mother. Fears are a normal part of parenting and all mothers experience them on occasion. So while these may seem like extreme parenting behaviours, as your confidence grows, many of these feelings will fade. If you find they are getting out of hand, your doctor can provide resources for helping you manage your anxiety.

Fear of SIDS

One of the most stressful fears for parents who have had a loss is the fear of SIDS, or Sudden Infant Death Syndrome. Much like stillbirth, SIDS can appear to strike out of nowhere. However, in one of the most successful public health campaigns in recent years, rates of SIDS have dropped in half since the introduction of Back to Sleep campaigns. If you're unfamiliar with the basics, remember the **ABCs**. Babies sleep safest **A**lone, on their **B**acks, in their **C**ribs. In my day job of teaching systematic review methods, the SIDS example is one of the most powerful. In a systematic review, a committee of several professionals reviews what is known in the research literature about a particular topic in a way that minimizes bias. They do this by setting out the criteria for including studies beforehand, developing a search of both the published and unpublished literature in a way that makes it more likely that they will find everything on a topic, and by combining all the studies together. These steps help to reduce the likelihood that a single biased study will influence the results. This allows them to make statements that can guide how medical professionals practice. In many cases, studies are done on a small scale, or on a specific group of people, and physicians are reluctant to change their practice in the face of limited proof. Once a systematic review demonstrated a clear benefit to showing that babies had a lower risk of SIDS if placed on their backs, public health campaigns were launched in Australia, Canada, the United Kingdom, and the United States to let both medical professionals and the general public know.

One systematic reviewer wanted to know not just what the best position was for a baby, but also how soon *we ought to have known* that back sleeping is best (78). After all, the first research published showing that back sleeping was best was done in 1944. Why did it take more than 50 years for that to become the common practice? So the researchers looked at the evidence in chronological order, to see how long it took before enough studies had been done to show clearly that one position was best. They found that as early as 1970, we should have been putting babies to sleep on their backs. I use this example for my nursing students to demonstrate the importance of keeping current with nursing research, of understanding how to read research papers, and of the value of systematic reviews. For parents with a fear of losing their child to SIDS, ensuring babies go to sleep on their backs is critical. As for being alone and in a crib, you can keep the crib in the same room as you to ease your mind about hearing them breathe and to make it easier to breastfeed. Despite all this, the first time they sleep through a feed, I guarantee you will be anxious about how they're doing. This is normal and natural. Crib alarms are not generally recommended (they are not foolproof) and bed sharing is controversial. For me, having my kids in my room, but out of my bed, was a good compromise.

Bonding with Your New Baby

While fairy tales may be filled with stories of love at first sight, for many of us, bonding is a lifelong process. As we grow and mature and change, just as our child grows and matures and changes, we will always be remaking and reforming our relationship. With each day you spend with your child, whether taking them to the park, reading them a story, or giving them a bath, you will be getting to know them better. You'll also be getting to know yourself better as a mother, and this is part of the bonding process. There is no single moment that you and your child are officially bonded. Escaping your own guilt over parenting behaviours is a helpful way to grow along with your child.

As your child grows, you will likely want to find ways to help them get to know their sibling who died and to incorporate your lost baby into the family. Many mothers see it as their job to ensure their lost babies are not forgotten. Telling your other children about their lost sibling is an important part of that remembrance process. As one mother said, "you can't have family secrets about big things—that would be the worst" (77).

That was certainly my own perception. If my children found out one day about their brothers from someone else, or by coming across my memory box for them, they would feel hurt and betrayed and confused. By making their brothers' existence simply part of the normal lives of our family, my children are better prepared for asking questions of me, either about their brothers or about death in general. Now that my daughter is older, we are asking her more about how she wants to honour them. She usually does this by making and decorating a cake, together with me. Many families involve the siblings on visits to the cemetery, or by attending memorial ceremonies and butterfly releases.

I started to introduce my daughter to her brothers by reading her a developmentally appropriate book when she was almost four years old, which was around the time of Nate and Sam's birthday. The book explained with simple words and pictures that there was a baby before she was born that died, and that even though the mommy and daddy in the story were sad sometimes, they were still very happy to have another child in their lives. Even though their ashes and a photo of them is in our bedroom, she has never asked to see the picture or wondered who was in the photo. At this time, her concept of them, and of death, remains very abstract. While there have been a couple of times she has been scared of death, I am not sure her fears are different from those of other four-year-olds. I answer her questions as she asks them. Certainly, this has led to some awkward moments. Last year she loudly announced to everyone in the YMCA change room that today was her brothers' birthday, and that "they're dead." I'm sure this caused a lot of moms to have some explaining to do to their own kids, but I can live with that.

There are many ways to honour your child who was lost and celebrate your child who has arrived. It is up to you what you do and how you do it. Watching your child grow and develop into a beautiful, confident, capable adult is the most wonderful gift of all.

12

JUST FOR FATHERS

> *To claim Irene I drove to a place that called itself a home. There I paid a man who called himself a mortician to hand over paperwork, along with what he called cremains. The ashes were stored in a cardboard box laminated with faux wood grain, like the vinyl paneling that adorns family recreation rooms and the flanks of station wagons. Inside the box was a gilded tin; inside the tin was a plastic bag closed at the top with a twist tie from which dangled a dog tag: "MONTROSE CEMETERY 27683."*
>
> *At home, I removed the baggie and threw out the box and tin. I slipped the dog tag into an envelope along with the death certificate—there was by law no birth certificate— licked the envelope, and sealed it. After a moment of deliberation, I filed the envelope under "Medical Bills." After another moment of deliberation, I made a new file folder— "Irene Raeburn"—slid the envelope in there, and filed it after "Investments." Then I wept. That was my fatherhood.*
>
> **—Daniel Raeburn in Vessels (79)**

Because You Are Expecting Too

Being pregnant after a loss is a challenging time for fathers, too. While we are getting better at acknowledging that men feel grief just as deeply as women do but express it differently, the truth is that the experience of men who have lost a child is not as well studied. I cannot provide you with tried and true tips, both because I am not a man and because the research is just not available. I can tell you that your job is to support your partner. But you also have to support your own mental health. Sometimes this is easy, and sometimes it can be very hard. Approximately ten percent of women who lose a baby go on to have a pregnancy with another partner. This means that you may not have ever experienced the death of a baby yourself, but still want to know how you can best support her during what is both an exciting and happy time for you and an anxious and difficult time for her. Regina describes how her husband, Scott, behaved during her pregnancy: "He's acting the same way as when I was pregnant with Jacob. He's worried, but he does not want to show it because he does not want me to be extra worried."

Needing to Be More Involved

A lot of men report feeling a need to be more involved in this pregnancy and a greater awareness that this pregnancy needs to be watched closely. This is not to suggest that you were not involved before, but certainly not every dad can attend every doctor's appointment. Maybe during your last pregnancy you felt more comfortable having her go on her own, or did not feel you could take the time off work. This time around, you might be feeling a greater sense that you need to be there, either to be vigilant in ensuring the doctor is doing his job, or to be able to have a closer look at the baby by going to every ultrasound. As one dad describes it, "I have made real special attempts to go with her every time she has been to the doctor. And those visits are times of anxiety. I've tried to be a lot more conscientious and careful, and you know, every doctor's visit I go with her and be there at those visits and things like that" (80).

---

15 Things I Need My Partner to Know During Our Pregnancy After Loss
June 22, 2014 by Lindsey Henke

1. I am scared, like really, really scared. I know now that things can go wrong and not every pregnancy has a happy ending. I really, really, really do not want lightning to strike twice, but I am afraid it will.

2. I need your support now more than ever. You are the only one who has been through this with me. So you are the only one who gets it like I do and because of that I need your support more than anyone else's.

3. I am confused because I am happy and joyful while full of grief and sadness all at the same time on top of fluctuating hormones, yes I am a mess and I need you to say that's okay.

4. Pregnancy after a loss is hard. I have post-traumatic stress disorder and anxiety, some days I get depressed and every day I am pregnant I am reliving my trauma on top of having the normal pregnancy stresses. Some say the closer I get to D-day (delivery that is), I'll feel better. Some say it gets worse, but I want you to know that there is no easy day for me right now.

5. I still miss the baby we lost. This one does not replace him/her. It actually makes all of this more difficult and painful.

6. I sometimes have trouble bonding with baby. I am scared to attach to him or her because I do not want my heart to get broken again. I sometimes catch myself creating a suit of armour around my heart as a way of protecting me from the pain that comes from loving and losing. I want you to know I do not want to be this way, it just happens from time to time as I try to protect myself from the fear of future heartache.

7. I am afraid I will not love this baby as much as our other one. I love our other child so much. My heart aches for him/her every day and because I yearn for our baby that is deceased with so much love I worry that there will not be enough love in my heart for our next one.

8. Sometimes I do not want to have sex as I worry that it might hurt the baby even though the doctor has reassured us this is not true.

9. I do not know how to handle this. I just do not. Pregnancy may not be new to me, but pregnancy after loss is. And it is just as new to me as much as it is to you. There is no road map, no right or wrong way to handle this balance of grief and joy. There is just messiness and beauty all smashed together during these nine months and I do not have the answers.

10. Please be patient with me as I am emotionally fragile, more fragile than I've ever been. I am super sensitive because my world was turned upside down when our baby died and our hopes and dreams died along with our child. My strength is all used up by the end of the day and my emotions are the hardest thing to keep in check. I hope you understand.

11. I have a hard time trusting my body as I feel like it has failed me before and I do not know how to believe in it now. I do not know how to trust my body or life. Life seems more unpredictable and fragile now and that scares me as I venture into carrying a new life inside of me again.

12. I am hopeful and grateful. I am hopeful that this baby is born ALIVE and healthy and lives a long beautiful life. I am also grateful that we were able to get pregnant again as I know many in our situation cannot and I am grateful for our baby that died. I know life is hard without him/her but I am glad he/she was here for a little while.

13. I just want pregnancy to be over with and for it to be frozen in this moment forever all at the same time. I want life, our baby's life, to be a sure thing, guaranteed. I am not trying to wish away this pregnancy. I just want to hold my breathing baby in my arms so I can be reassured everything will be okay this time.

14. I want so badly to bring this baby safely into the world for you, for me, for our baby that died, for our healing, for us, and there is a lot of pressure on me because I want it so bad. I do not want to feel like I let you down again even though I know I never did.

15. I love you and I need you to love me and this baby unconditionally. Because that is the only way I believe we will get through these nine months, by holding onto each other in hopes of someday soon holding onto our breathing baby.

Extra:
16. I know if I had to I could do this without you, but I do not want to. Pregnancy after loss is hard, but it is easier to get through each day with you by my side.

Having an advocate at your side when you go to a doctor's appointment is a good idea for anyone. If you are able to take time off from work and go with your partner, it can be a great experience for both of you. You can help her by remembering any questions she might have, and by not being afraid to ask a few of your own. Ask the doctor, midwife, or nurse if there are specific things you can do to help.

But sometimes, your trying to help can feel a little suffocating for your partner, especially because she may already be feeling a lack of self-confidence during this pregnancy. Even if you have never done anything to make her feel that way, she may be worried that you blame her for the death of your last child and worry that you do not trust her to be capable to birth this baby alive either. So take your cues for involvement from her.

Taking a tour of the hospital, even if you have been there before, can be very helpful. Jenn describes the tour she took with her husband Lucas:

> "We were at the hospital on Friday on a tour of the postnatal ward. They are in the same part of the building as the antenatal ward. He was feeling quite anxious about being there and looking the same as the antenatal ward where we found out Fiona had died. They offered to show us around and that was helpful and it meant going back to the labour suite, which was the first time he has been back there since we left without Fiona. I have been back loads of times, but that was very emotional for him. Lucas was really tense when we were back in the room that we had been in. I think that is a very emotional journey for him. He just deals with it a little bit differently a lot of the time."

Coping with Anxiety and Stress

Anxiety and stress are very common for both mothers and fathers in the pregnancy after a loss. If you are feeling it, learning how to cope and manage those feelings can be beneficial to both of you. One of the most stressful times can be the ultrasound appointments. Because this is often when parents first discover that their child has died, going back to the same hospital or clinic, to the same room where you experienced that horrible news, can bring flashbacks and uncomfortable feelings. The sights, smells, sounds, and experience can seem so similar, even when you logically know that this time, things are different. One dad described himself as being "scared to death. That's the worst part. Waiting to see her move or hearing the doctor say it is okay. They do not say anything at eight weeks. ...It is pretty stressful that first couple of minutes. That's how we found out Mary had died. We went to that level II, and she had...we saw there is no heartbeat. So that's why I am so scared of ultrasounds" (52).

If anxiety over ultrasounds is an issue for you, acknowledging that this can be a challenging experience can be a good start in conquering the anxiety. While the fetal assessment clinic should be aware or your past history, you can phone them ahead of time to ensure they give you extra consideration, such as making sure they measure the baby's heart rate first. Research is not clear as to whether fathers feel as much anxiety as mothers, or if their anxiety wanes as the baby get closer to delivery. There is also some suggestion that for couples that get pregnant quickly, less anxiety is felt by fathers than those in couples that take some time to get pregnant (12).

Again, with limited research it is hard to know what to prepare for or how to cope. In any case, I believe forewarned is forearmed, and simply knowing that you are not the first father to experience higher stress levels during a pregnancy after a loss can help. Steph talks about how important communicating about the stress was with her husband, Chris. Together they made sure to touch base with one another about whatever emotions they were feeling, as a way to manage the pressure felt from outside their marriage. As she says, "My marriage has gotten stronger for it because I know it is something that can totally tear a family apart. I think that we were lucky in the fact that we just grew stronger as friends and as a couple. We both agreed to be very open about it. Talking about his anger and stuff like that. It was great because that was how I wanted it to be. I did not want it to just be this sad thing that happened that we put behind us."

Developing healthy coping strategies can be critical to making things easier for your partner, too. Many men report drinking more in the months following their stillbirth, or using illicit drugs. Only about half of fathers received some sort of professional help, whether that was from a hospital social worker, a priest, pastor or other religious leader, or from their family doctor (12). However, 40 percent of fathers reported wishing they had had more help in the form of further support. Seeking out professional advice can be beneficial to both you and your partner.

Bonding with Baby

Bonding with your baby before he or she is born is already a little tricky for fathers. Because you do not have the immediate experience of feeling the baby move or the physical changes of pregnancy reminding you of what is going on, it can be difficult to get the sense that your baby is real. When your previous pregnancy resulted in a loss, it can be extra challenging. Whether you are steeling yourself emotionally or are trying to be extra cautious, you may not feel ready to try to bond with this baby. But in bonding with your baby, and with your partner, you can be a great support to her.

These actions can also help relieve some of your anxiety. Here are some ideas that may help you. Try the ones that work for you, and maybe be inspired to think of some of your own.

1. Read to your baby. This is probably the most popular because it does not require any special equipment, other than a book! You can read any time day or night (your baby does not care). Books for babies can be obtained freely at the library or borrowed from friends. And even if the baby cannot really understand your words, reading to your partner's belly gets the baby used to hearing the sound of your voice. And even if you feel a little ridiculous reading about hungry caterpillars or barnyard dances, your kid will love it when daddy gets a little silly. But why should you read to them in utero? Mostly so you can get into the practice. Try and imagine what their response will be. Will your son love it when you roar like a dinosaur? Will he insist on reading Goodnight Moon just one more time before bed? Having these dreams about the future will help connect you to your baby in the here and now, especially if you have been holding yourself back this time around.

2. Be the family archivist/historian. Your partner may not be ready to obsessively mark every milestone in the baby book, just because she's not emotionally ready to go there yet. If you are, pull out a notebook or your iPhone and start recording things you will want to keep for a future baby book. When did she feel the first kicks? Write it down! What dates were the ultrasound appointments, and how was your partner feeling? You can write as much or as little as you feel comfortable with, but, by appointing yourself for this task, you will take some pressure off your spouse. This can be particularly helpful if you are excited about baby but she's not yet ready to tell the world.

3. Listen to the baby's heartbeat. If you are using a Doppler, you can help your partner use it and find comfort in hearing the heartbeat for yourself. Using the Doppler can increase anxiety for some people, so discuss with your partner if this is the right option for you. It can be a great source of reassurance when you are far enough along in the pregnancy to be able to pick up a heartbeat reliably but not far enough along to rely on kick counting.

4. Count the kicks. If your partner is doing kick counting, either using an app or a bracelet or just a piece of paper, join her in counting the movements. If you can, lie down beside her in the evening and place your hands on her belly. Spend a half hour lying peacefully, reading or watching television, or just talking, and make a mark in your app or on paper every time you feel a movement. See how many movements you feel compared with how many she feels. Another kick-counting game: put a coin on your partner's belly and see how many movements before the baby kicks it off.

5. Prepare the nursery. You might want to do this just before baby gets here, but you can do it whenever you feel ready. Because a lot of people find that working with their hands helps them to work through their grief, building something (even if it is just flat-pack furniture) can be a positive experience and help you to see this baby as something tangible. Whether you paint the room, put together a crib, or just take baby things bought for your last baby out of their storage boxes, all of these activities will help lessen the burden on your partner.

Whatever you choose, bonding with your baby can be difficult at this stage, so do not be too hard on yourself. Do what comes naturally and do not feel you have to push it.

Pregnancy After a Loss Is Hard on Your Marriage

There is no way around it: this can be a stressful time for your relationship. It is easy to think that once you have overcome the hurdle of initial grief, having a real, live baby would be the easy part. It is not. Much like when you first lost your child, your emotions can be wildly different from your partner's. You can blame what sex we are for this, and some of that is true, but the reality is that no two people experience grief in exactly the same way. Our sex shapes our response, but so does our religion, our culture, our relationships with others, our personality types, and so much more. Above all, your partner needs you to know that you support her. You will need to let her know that often.

Maeve talks about how important her husband, Gavin, was in supporting her through her emotions, and vice versa. "Gavin has gotten really excellent at supporting me when I am angry with people." She describes how he listened and commiserated when she had a difficult encounter with a friend who was not very understanding about how upset she was around the anniversary of the death of their baby. Being pregnant again after a loss has really changed their marriage, and while they have always worked together, since the death of their baby they have become closer. As she said, "This last year, we have done more together, whereas before we were fairly independent of each other. But now, any opportunity we have to take a trip together or do something and have lunch together, we try and do that. I used to just be in the office and be happy to do my own thing, and if he did not need me to come with him, I wouldn't." As she approaches the birth, she says, "Now, I do not want Gavin to be that far away from me. When we work (outside the office) I do not think I want him to be more than ten minutes away from me. Because Gavin is a huge support to me, emotionally and physically. As strange as that sounds, just to have him nearby and to know that if we have to go to the hospital that he will be able to come with me."

Finally, sex will be difficult. For a lot of men, sex helps them to bond with their partners, it helps them to feel connected. But both you and she may be fearful of what could happen. If either of you is not in the mood, the sex either will not happen at all, or it will not be very good. I do not have a magic solution to this problem, but knowing it is coming can help you work it through.

Once Baby Is Here

Again, you might be hoping for a huge wave of relief once you have a live baby in your arms. That from here on in, it will be nothing but sunshine and rainbows. Sorry to burst your bubble, but despite the incredible, overwhelming joy you will feel that first time you hold your baby in your arms...it will not last. Psychiatrists used to worry about something called the replacement child syndrome, where a baby born after a loss had unrealistic expectations placed on them. But like any other baby, this baby will not sleep through the night, will not always feed easily, will have explosive diapers, and miserable crying jags that seem to last until your ears bleed. In short, this baby will not be perfect. The stress of having your lives turned upside down still happens to couples who have undergone a loss. You will have to go to work in a daze, having been unable to sleep. If you did manage to sleep, your partner might spend all breakfast giving you the stink eye because she was up all night. You will feel hopelessly frustrated as no amount of rocking, cuddling, cooing, singing, or whatever other tricks you have up your sleeve, will calm your baby.

And worse, it seems to last forever. But the truth is, it does not. Think of it this way: If you got married at 30 and live to be 90, that's 60 years you get to spend with your wife. Even if as many as three whole years are miserable, that still means your marriage is happy 95 percent of the time! And, even if it feels like an eternity, it will not be three years. One evening, when you least expect it, you will put your baby down to bed and not fall asleep yourself immediately afterwards. You will surprise yourself when it happens, but it will. As Maeve describes it: "For so many first-time parents, parenthood wasn't what they expected it to be. I think their relationships have really changed and how they deal with their child's birth really changes them."

There are lots of ways fathers can help in those first few months of baby's arrival. From groceries and cooking, to laundry and dishes, to changing and playing with the baby, men can do everything but breastfeed. It can be really hard if you have a long commute, or work shifts, but try to do as much as you think you can.

Postpartum Support International is a great organization with resources to help. With offices in 42 countries, they offer help and support near you, in your language. They can be reached at:

(800)944–4PPD, (800)944–4773
http://www.postpartum.net

Postpartum Depression

No article on the reality of life with a new baby would be complete without a mention of postpartum depression. Of course, knowing where the line is between postpartum depression, plain old regular depression, and normal grief is tricky, and actually rather arbitrary. According to the Department of Health and Human Services in the US, about 13 percent of new mothers experience postpartum depression [81]. Numerous studies have found that women who have experienced a pregnancy loss are at higher risk of having postpartum depression [74, 82, 83]. You may not realize that fathers can experience postpartum depression too. Rates of postpartum depression in men are estimated to be similar to those for women, but much less researched and talked about [84].

Here are some questions to think about to determine if you might be having postpartum depression:

1. Are you withdrawing or avoiding things, such as social situations, work, or family?
2. Do you feel indecisive? Overly cynical? Angry? Incredibly irritated?
3. Do you feel emotionally anything at all?
4. Are you feeling very self-critical?
5. Have you been using more drugs or alcohol?
6. Do you find yourself fighting with your partner more?
7. Are you experiencing physical symptoms, such as indigestion, changes in appetite and weight, diarrhea, constipation, headache, toothache, nausea, and insomnia?
8. Are you concerned you are not becoming the father you want to be, maybe by using too many negative parenting behaviours (such as not enough warmth or sensitivity and too much hostility or disengagement)? (84)

If you are at all concerned that either your or your partner might be suffering from postpartum depression, find help! This can come in many forms, from asking your family doctor or a public health nurse or your midwife. There is no need to feel guilty, ashamed, or embarrassed about postpartum depression. It is incredibly common and not a sign that you are a bad father or partner. There are many different treatments for postpartum depression, from medications to talk therapy. Finding the right one for you is critical, which is why it needs to start with a consultation from a professional. Of course, the same goes if you witness these behaviours or emotions in your partner.

Pregnancy after a loss is a challenging time for both mothers and fathers. It is a time of transitions and changes and highs and lows. Together with your partner, you can make this one of the greatest times of your life. Jenn describes how life has changed now that Evelyn has been born. "To be clear with everybody, this does not fix everything. It is amazing to have a baby at home, and she is incredible, but it hasn't fixed anything. I read somewhere that having another baby does not make the loss better, but it does make life better. It is true. Evelyn hasn't made our loss any better, but she has made our life richer and amazing. There is loss, and there is life as well, and they are intertwined."

REFERENCES

1. Ahman E, Zupan J, World Health Organization. Dept. of Making Pregnancy Safer. Neonatal and perinatal mortality : country, regional and global estimates. Geneva: World Health Organization; 2007. Contract No.: Report.

2. Mills TA, Ricklesford C, Cooke A, Heazell AE, Whitworth M, Lavender T. Parents' experiences and expectations of care in pregnancy after stillbirth or neonatal death: a metasynthesis. BJOG: An International Journal of Obstetrics & Gynaecology. 2014;121(8):943-50.

3. Peters MD, Lisy K, Riitano D, Jordan Z, Aromataris E. Providing meaningful care for families experiencing stillbirth: a meta-synthesis of qualitative evidence. Journal of perinatology : official journal of the California Perinatal Association. 2016;36(1):3-9.

4. American College of Obstetricians and Gynecologists. ACOG Practice bulletin no. 115: Vaginal birth after previous cesarean delivery. Obstetrics and gynecology. 2010;116(2, part 1):450-63.

5. Royal College of Obstetricians and Gynaecologists. Birth After Previous Caesarean Birth. 2007. p. 1-17.

6. Gold KJ, Leon I, Chames MC. National survey of obstetrician attitudes about timing the subsequent pregnancy after perinatal death. American Journal of Obstetrics & Gynecology. 2010;202(4):357.e1-.e6.

7. Bhattacharya S, Smith N. Pregnancy following miscarriage: what is the optimum interpregnancy interval? Women's health. 2011;7(2):139-41.

8. Conde-Agudelo A, Rosas-Bermudez A, Kafury-Goeta AC. Birth spacing and risk of adverse perinatal outcomes: a meta-analysis. JAMA. 2006;295(15):1809-23.

9. Reid M. The experience of babies born following the loss of a baby. In: Urwin C, Sternberg J, editors. Infant observation and research: emotional processes in everyday lives. Hove, East Sussex ; New York: Routledge; 2012. p. 123-34.

10. Oxford English Dictionary. "penumbra, n.": Oxford University Press.

11. Kübler-Ross E. On death and dying. Electronic reproduction. UK : MyiLibrary ed. London: Tavistock/Routledge; 1989 1970.

12. Turton P, Badenhorst W, Hughes P, Ward J, Riches S, White S. Psychological impact of stillbirth on fathers in the subsequent pregnancy and puerperium. Journal of Mental Science. 2006;188(2):165-72.

13. Wilcox AJ, Weinberg CR, Baird DD. Timing of sexual intercourse in relation to ovulation. Effects on the probability of conception, survival of the pregnancy, and sex of the baby. New England Journal of Medicine. 1995;333(23):1517-21.

14. Cunningham FG. Williams obstetrics. 24th edition. ed. New York: McGraw-Hill Education/Medical; 2014. xviii, 1358 pages p.

15. Natural Medicine. Fertility Type Conditions Monograph [Database]. Therapeutic Research Center. 2016 [cited August 19, 2016].

16. James U. Practical uses of clinical hypnosis in enhancing fertility, healthy pregnancy and childbirth. Complementary Therapies in Clinical Practice. 2009;15(4):239-41.

17. Galhardo A, Cunha M, Pinto-Gouveia J. Mindfulness-Based Program for Infertility: efficacy study. Fertility & Sterility. 2013;100(4):1059-67.

18. Schuurmans N, Senikas V, Lalonde AB. Healthy Beginnings: Giving your baby the best start, from preconception to birth. Mississauga: Wiley; 2009.

19. Showell MG, Mackenzie-Proctor R, Brown J, Yazdani A, Stankiewicz MT, Hart RJ. Antioxidants for male subfertility. Cochrane Database of Systematic Reviews. 2014;12:CD007411.

20. Safarinejad MR, Safarinejad S. Efficacy of selenium and/or N-acetyl-cysteine for improving semen parameters in infertile men: a double-blind, placebo controlled, randomized study. Journal of Urology. 2009;181(2):741-51.

21. Mistry HD, Broughton Pipkin F, Redman CW, Poston L. Selenium in reproductive health. American Journal of Obstetrics & Gynecology. 2012;206(1):21-30.

22. Showell MG, Brown J, Clarke J, Hart RJ. Antioxidants for female subfertility. Cochrane Database of Systematic Reviews. 2013;8:007807.

23. Westphal LM, Polan ML, Trant AS. Double-blind, placebo-controlled study of Fertilityblend: a nutritional supplement for improving fertility in women. Clinical & Experimental Obstetrics & Gynecology. 2006;33(4):205-8.

24. Lim CE, Ng RW, Xu K, Cheng NC, Xue CC, Liu JP, et al. Acupuncture for polycystic ovarian syndrome. Cochrane Database of Systematic Reviews. 2016(5):CD007689.

25. Anderson K, Norman RJ, Middleton P. Preconception lifestyle advice for people with subfertility. Cochrane Database of Systematic Reviews. 2010(4):008189.

26. Sharma R, Biedenharn KR, Fedor JM, Agarwal A. Lifestyle factors and reproductive health: taking control of your fertility. Reproductive Biology & Endocrinology.

2013;11:66.

27. McLean M, Wellons MF. Optimizing natural fertility: the role of lifestyle modification. Obstetrics & Gynecology Clinics of North America. 2012;39(4):465-77.

28. Martinez-Palomo A. Revisiting Zika (and Rubella). Journal of public health policy. 2016.

29. Cote-Arsenault DMR. One foot in-one foot out: weathering the storm of pregnancy after perinatal loss. Research in Nursing and Health. 2000;23(6):473-85.

30. Sandall J, Soltani H, Gates S, Shennan A, Devane D. Midwife-led continuity models versus other models of care for childbearing women. Cochrane Database of Systematic Reviews. 2016;4:CD004667.

31. Sackett DL, Rosenberg WM, Gray JA, Haynes RB, Richardson WS. Evidence based medicine: what it is and what it isn't. BMJ. 1996;312(7023):71-2.

32. Makrydimas G, Sebire NJ, Lolis D, Vlassis N, Nicolaides KH. Fetal loss following ultrasound diagnosis of a live fetus at 6-10 weeks of gestation. Ultrasound in Obstetrics & Gynecology. 2003;22(4):368-72.

33. Tong S, Kaur A, Walker SP, Bryant V, Onwude JL, Permezel M. Miscarriage risk for asymptomatic women after a normal first-trimester prenatal visit. Obstetrics & Gynecology. 2008;111(3):710-4.

34. Cedergren M, Brynhildsen J, Josefsson A, Sydsjo A, Sydsjo G. Hyperemesis gravidarum that requires hospitalization and the use of antiemetic drugs in relation to maternal body composition. American Journal of Obstetrics & Gynecology. 2008;198(4):412.e1-.e5.

35. Veenendaal MV, van Abeelen AF, Painter RC, van der Post JA, Roseboom TJ. Consequences of hyperemesis gravidarum for offspring: a systematic review and meta-analysis. BJOG: An International Journal of Obstetrics & Gynaecology. 2011;118(11):1302-13.

36. Natural Medicines. Nausea and vomiting. Natural Medicines Bottom Line Monograph: Natural Medicines; 2016.

37. Kong JS, Teuber SS, Gershwin ME. Aspirin and nonsteroidal anti-inflammatory drug hypersensitivity. Clinical reviews in allergy & immunology. 2007;32(1):97-110.

38. Ross LE, Grigoriadis S, Mamisashvili L, Vonderporten EH, Roerecke M, Rehm J, et al. Selected pregnancy and delivery outcomes after exposure to antidepressant medication: a systematic review and meta-analysis. JAMA Psychiatry. 2013;70(4):436-43.

39. Doubilet PM, Benson CB. Atlas of ultrasound in obstetrics and gynecology.

Philadelphia: Wolters Kluwer/Lippincott Williams & Wilkins Health; 2012. p. 432.

40. Cote-Arsenault D, Donato KL, Earl SS. Watching & worrying: Early pregnancy after loss experiences. MCN: The American Journal of Maternal/Child Nursing. 2006;31(6):356-63.

41. Cote-Arsenault D, Freije MM. Support groups helping women through pregnancies after loss. Western journal of nursing research. 2004;26(6):650-70.

42. Scanlon VC, Sanders T. Essentials of anatomy and physiology. Philadelphia, PA: F.A. Davis Co.; 2011. p. 640.

43. Salvesen K, Lees C, Abramowicz J, Brezinka C, Ter Haar G, Marsal K, et al. ISUOG statement on the safe use of Doppler in the 11 to 13 +6-week fetal ultrasound examination. Ultrasound in Obstetrics & Gynecology. 2011;37(6):628.

44. Blackburn ST. Maternal, fetal, & neonatal physiology: a clinical perspective. St. Louis, Mo.: Saunders Elsevier; 2007. 777 p.

45. Zieve D, Eltz DR. Chorionic villus sampling 2014 [updated Nov. 16, 2014. Available from: https://medlineplus.gov/ency/article/003406.htm.

46. Wittels KA, Pelletier AJ, Brown DF, Camargo CA, Jr. United States emergency department visits for vaginal bleeding during early pregnancy, 1993-2003. American Journal of Obstetrics & Gynecology. 2008;198(5):523.e1-.e6.

47. Mason MC. Help at last for women who lose babies. Nursing Standard. 2010;25(3):24-5.

48. Musters AM, Taminiau-Bloem EF, van den Boogaard E, van der Veen F, Goddijn M. Supportive care for women with unexplained recurrent miscarriage: patients' perspectives. Human Reproduction. 2011;26(4):873-7.

49. Sugiura-Ogasawara M, Nakano Y, Ozaki Y, Furukawa TA. Possible improvement of depression after systematic examination and explanation of live birth rates among women with recurrent miscarriage. Journal of Obstetrics & Gynaecology. 2013;33(2):171-4.

50. Mortensen LL, Hegaard HK, Andersen AN, Bentzen JG. Attitudes towards motherhood and fertility awareness among 20-40-year-old female healthcare professionals. European Journal of Contraception & Reproductive Health Care. 2012;17(6):468-81.

51. KidsHealth from Nemours. Week by Week Pregnancy Calendar 2016 [updated August 2016. 2016:[Available from: http://kidshealth.org/en/parents/pregnancy-calendar-intro.html.

52. O'Leary J. The trauma of ultrasound during a pregnancy following perinatal loss. Journal of Loss and Trauma. 2005;10(2):183-204.

53. Sacks DN. Amniocentesis: MedlinePlus Medical Encyclopedia 2015 [cited 2016 Sept 21, 2016]. Available from: https://medlineplus.gov/ency/article/003921.htm.

54. Royal College of Obstetricians and Gynaecologists. Amniocentesis and chorionic villus sampling. 2010. Greentop Guideline No 8: Report.

55. Locock L, Field K, McPherson A, Boyd PA. Women's accounts of the physical sensation of chorionic villus sampling and amniocentesis: expectations and experience. Midwifery. 2010;26(1):64-75.

56. Van Schoubroeck D, Verhaeghe J. Does local anesthesia at mid-trimester amniocentesis decrease pain experience? A randomized trial in 220 patients. Ultrasound in Obstetrics and Gynecology. 2000;16(6):536-8.

57. Venes D, Taber CW. Taber's cyclopedic medical dictionary. Philadelphia: F.A. Davis; 2013. 2846 p.

58. The Name Lady. After the Loss of a Child, Can I Still Have a Junior? 2011 [cited 2011]. Available from: http://www.namecandy.com/name-lady/2011/11/28/after-the-loss-of-a-child-can-i-still-have-a-junior.

59. Mennella JA, Jagnow CP, Beauchamp GK. Prenatal and postnatal flavor learning by human infants. Pediatrics. 2001;107(6):E88.

60. Murkoff HE, Eisenberg A, Hathaway SE. What to expect when you're expecting. New York: Workman Pub.; 2002. 597 p.

61. National Center for Immunization and Respiratory Diseases. Get Whooping Cough Vaccine While You Are Pregnant 2014 [Available from: http://www.cdc.gov/vaccines/adults/rec-vac/pregnant/whooping-cough/get-vaccinated.html.

62. Blakeslee S. The CRAAP Test. LOEX Quarterly. 2004;31:6-7.

63. Reece EA, Barbieri RL. Obstetrics and gynecology : the essentials of clinical care. Reece EA, Barbieri RL, editors. Stuttgart ; New York: Thieme; 2010. xv, 557 p. : ill. p.

64. Whitworth MK, Fisher M, Heazell AE, Royal College of Obstetricians and Gynaecologists. Reduced fetal movements: Green Top Guideline No. 57. Royal College of Obstetricians and Gynaecologists; 2011.

65. Maser S. Blessingways: A Guide to Mother-Centred Baby Showers - Celebrating Pregnancy, Birth, and Motherhood. Ann Arbor, MI: Moondance Press; 2004.

66. Coyle ME, Smith CA, Peat B. Cephalic version by moxibustion for breech

presentation. The Cochrane database of systematic reviews. 2012;5:CD003928.

67. American College of Obstetricians and Gynecologists. External Cephalic Version (Version) for Breech Position: FAQ 079: ACOG; 2015 [updated April 2015. Available from: http://www.acog.org/Patients/FAQs/If-Your-Baby-Is-Breech.

68. Robson SJ, Leader LR. Management of subsequent pregnancy after an unexplained stillbirth. Journal of Perinatology. 2010;30(5):305-10.

69. AWHONN. 40 Reasons to Go the Full 40 Weeks. 2012. Available from: http://www. health4mom.org/zones/go-the-full-40

70. Kozhimannil KB, Macheras M, Lorch SA. Trends in childbirth before 39 weeks' gestation without medical indication. Medical care. 2014;52(7):649-57.

71. Taber CW, Venes D, Stat!Ref, Teton Data S. Taber's cyclopedic medical dictionary. Philadelphia: F.A. Davis; 2013.

72. O'Leary JM. The baby who follows the loss of a sibling: special considerations in the postpartum period. International Journal of Childbirth Education. 2005;20(4):28-30.

73. Gavin NI, Gaynes BN, Lohr KN, Meltzer-Brody S, Gartlehner G, Swinson T. Perinatal depression: a systematic review of prevalence and incidence. Obstetrics & Gynecology. 2005;106(5 Pt 1):1071-83.

74. Giannandrea SAM, Cerulli C, Anson E, Chaudron LH. Increased Risk for Postpartum Psychiatric Disorders Among Women with Past Pregnancy Loss. Journal of Women's Health (15409996). 2013;22(9):760-8.

75. Moretti M. Breastfeeding and the use of antidepressants. Journal of Population Therapeutics & Clinical Pharmacology. 2012;19(3):e387-90.

76. Lamb EH. The impact of previous perinatal loss on subsequent pregnancy and parenting. Journal of Perinatal Education. 2002;11(2):33-40.

77. Cote-Arsenault D. Weaving babies lost in pregnancy into the fabric of the family. Journal of Family Nursing. 2003;9(1):23-37.

78. Gilbert R, Salanti G, Harden M, See S. Infant sleeping position and the sudden infant death syndrome: systematic review of observational studies and historical review of recommendations from 1940 to 2002. International journal of epidemiology. 2005;34(4):874-87.

79. Raeburn D. Vessels. The New Yorker. 2006:48-53.

80. Armstrong D. Exploring fathers' experiences of pregnancy after a prior perinatal loss. MCN - American Journal of Maternal Child Nursing. 2001;26(3):147-53.

81. US Department of Health and Human Services Office on Women's Health. Depression during and after pregnancy fact sheet Washington, DC: US Department of Health and Human Services, Office on Womens Health; 2016 [updated February 12, 2016; cited 2016 October 27, 2016]. Available from: https://www.womenshealth.gov/publications/our-publications/fact-sheet/depression-pregnancy.html.

82. Hunfeld JA, Taselaar-Kloos AK, Agterberg G, Wladimiroff JW, Passchier J. Trait anxiety, negative emotions, and the mothers' adaptation to an infant born subsequent to late pregnancy loss: a case-control study. Prenatal diagnosis. 1997;17(9):843-51.

83. Blackmore ER, Cote-Arsenault D, Tang W, Glover V, Evans J, Golding J, et al. Previous prenatal loss as a predictor of perinatal depression and anxiety. British Journal of Psychiatry. 2011;198(5):373-8.

84. Musser AK, Ahmed AH, Foli KJ, Coddington JA. Paternal postpartum depression: what health care providers should know. Journal of Pediatric Health Care. 2013;27(6):479-85.

About the Author

Amanda Ross-White is the proud mother of four beautiful children, including her twin boys Nate and Sam, who were stillborn in 2007. She is eternally grateful to watch her rainbow children, daughter Rebecca and son Alex, grow around her. Since joining the sad world of the babylost, she has become dedicated to furthering research into stillbirth and neonatal death, as well as the unique parenting and relationship challenges for babylost mothers. In her day job, she helps connect people to the medical and health information they need, and sees the need for better communication between babylost mothers and their health care providers. She graduated in 2002 from Western University with her MLIS and in 2000 from McGill University. Since 2004, she has worked at Queen's University as the Nursing Librarian, where she teaches information literacy to both undergraduate and postgraduate nursing students. Her research interests are on systematic reviews and the searching, retrieval and evaluation of research literature.